Acknowledgments

Thank you to my husband, Mitch, and son, Derek. You were the first to believe in and encourage me to go for it. Your support and enthusiasm for this project gave me the confidence to keep at it. It is wonderful to have you as my greatest fans.

To Joan Donovan, my fabulous editor, I am in awe of how you take my words and turn them into just what my heart wants to say. I have learned so much from you. Thank you for your guidance, patience, and great sense of humor.

Thank you to Dan Chin and Steve Busalacchi, who advised, encouraged, and connected me with the right people throughout the entire process.

Thank you to my coworkers at Agrace HospiceCare, who have answered the call with such dedication. The care and compassion you demonstrate every day inspires me.

Most important, thank you to the patients and their families served by Agrace HospiceCare. You teach us so much … before you go.

Before You Go

Published by CMD Presents, LLC
Madison, WI

All rights reserved
Copyright 2013 by Cheri Milton

Cover design by Ryan Perkins
Back cover photo by Wesley Peck
Book design by Jason Warholic

ISBN 978-0-9886938-0-7

BEFORE YOU GO

Contents

i	Acknowledgments
v	Introduction
1	At Least I Can Still …: *Joyce*
11	Advice from a Purple Poodle: *Lily*
21	Holding on … and Letting Go: *Mary*
33	Don't Wait, Open Your Gifts: *Harold*
43	When Truth Can Shatter: *Shirley*
57	'Say What You Need to Say': *Eric*
69	Ghosts Shadowing Ghosts: *Ricky*
81	Just Be There: *Marvin*
89	Growing Wings in Freefall: *Lori*
99	We're Built for Overcoming: *Liz*
111	Peace, Only Peace: *Bob*
121	Close to Home: *Carson*

BEFORE YOU GO

Introduction

When I started working with hospice patients almost seven years ago, I knew I was blessed to find such meaningful work. Like many in this field, I felt called to it. I was ready to do my part to fulfill our mission: Enhancing the Quality of Life at the End of Life. Eagerly I met patients and their families to offer what help I could give.

Quite often I would arrive home and relay the day's events to my husband and son as we sat around the dinner table. Hearing how moved I was working with patients and families, they would respond, "You need to write these stories down!"

And so I began to keep a journal, making entries on the days I was most deeply affected, even rocked, by my patients' struggles, triumphs, and tragedies. From those journal entries, *Before You Go* evolved.

To this day, the honor and privilege of coming into my patients' lives, homes, and families as they face their final days are powerful and sacred. Their pain, courage, and humanity have taught me so much about what truly matters in life, and I am forever changed.

The twelve stories in these pages are some of the most memorable patient and family situations I have encountered. They are true accounts of what I experienced in my work; however, all identifying details have been changed to ensure the privacy of the individuals and families involved.

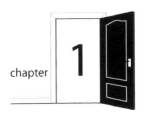

Joyce

BEFORE YOU GO

At Least I Can Still …

Where is a wise man who does not grieve for the things which he has not, but rejoices for those which he has.

Epictetus

We all have them, those days that just don't go well. Actually, I was having one of those weeks. Monday was not even minimally close to plan but full of interruptions and unanticipated tasks. Tuesday rolled out with a vengeance, hot coffee spilling all over my desk—including my computer keyboard. No one to blame there but myself!

Soon enough I discovered that I'd forgotten my work phone at home. By 9 a.m. I was dully aware that my new shoes were already hurting my feet.

But my mood went to lip-curling black when the fat stack of papers I dropped by the copier went skipping and scattering down the hallway in front of my peers. Couldn't I just go back home? Shouldn't I?

My irritation at these minor events soon spiraled down into a repetitive lament about how tired I was, how overwhelmed I felt. Two days shot already—I'm going to be behind the whole rest of the week! My thoughts were simmering just below a boil when the phone rang, snapping me back to the present.

"Are you busy today?" It was Ann, our hospice social worker. "Any chance you could meet with Joyce Schmidt, my new ALS patient?"

I took a deep breath. Ann rushed to tell me she'd already informed Joyce and her family about my role as grief counselor on her care team.

Her voice grew excited. "Cherí, when she heard about your part, Joyce just jumped at the chance to talk with you. She'd really like to see you right away—today, if possible. What do you think?"

Reflexively I did a quick review of what was on my calendar for the afternoon. It was possible, yes, but I was worn out! Sighing to myself, and grateful that Ann couldn't see my grimace, I answered, "Yes, I can do it." Seeing a patient who has an expressed need takes priority and automatically resets the schedule for my day, regardless.

We set a time of 1 p.m. Ann would call the family to confirm.

One o'clock found me crossing the threshold into Joyce Schmidt's world. She sat waiting for me, wheelchair-bound, on the other side of an expansive family room adjoining the kitchen. A nursing assistant was putting her socks on for her.

The room offered two large, bright-colored couches and multiple plush chairs to welcome the many friends and neighbors who wanted to visit or help out in some way. Joyce and her husband, Carl, had attracted a network of constant support through many years of community involvement.

The Schmidts had carefully remodeled their home to allow Joyce to move about the main floor with ease. A ground-level master bedroom had been added the year before, in expectation of the day when carrying Joyce upstairs would be unmanageable for her caregivers.

Except for the daily newspaper in disarray on the floor, all was tidy. Several family members, including Joyce's daughter,

Amy, and a close friend of Joyce's, buzzed around the kitchen doing dishes left over from breakfast and lunch. From time to time during my visit, the clatter of dishes going into the dishwasher punctuated the low hum of kitchen conversation. A lively energy pervaded the home.

Despite her advanced ALS, Joyce was still able to lift her head. She tilted a bright, alert face toward me and smiled slightly, inviting me to sit down. I took a seat facing her and smiled back. Her still-pretty face was framed by loose natural curls of a cinnamon color, only slightly touched by gray. What a blessing to have such a naturally lovely color and curl! It struck me that Joyce must have been the envy of her girlfriends in her younger days.

The nursing assistant was finishing up for the day—having completed a regimen of personal care for Joyce that included administering her daily bath, drying her hair, and dressing her. Her shampoo smelled of green apple and made me aware of being a little bit hungry. I considered that it was probably not having the same effect on Joyce, who received all her nourishment from a feeding tube these days. The life-stealing effects of ALS were all too apparent. Joyce could not eat or speak or move her body.

Indeed, I was acutely aware that Joyce had only diminished capacity ahead of her. The ALS Association offers this precise, and horrifying, description of the fatal course of the disease:

> Amyotrophic lateral sclerosis (ALS), often referred to as "Lou Gehrig's Disease," is a progressive neurodegenerative disease that affects nerve cells in the brain and the spinal cord. Motor neurons reach from the brain to the spinal cord and from the spinal cord to the muscles throughout the body. The progressive degeneration of the motor neurons in ALS eventually leads to death. When the motor neurons die, the ability

of the brain to initiate and control muscle movement is lost. With voluntary muscle action progressively affected, patients in the later stages of the disease may become totally paralyzed.

In other words, this disease just keeps taking away. At the very end the patient is left struggling to breathe. Could there be a more cruel death sentence?

※ ※ ※

After the nursing assistant had wrapped up and said a pleasant goodbye to us, Joyce and I sat together alone. With muscles stuttering and jerking, she slowly lifted her head and steadied her gaze toward me. Using only her expressive face and a distinctive raising of her eyebrows, she clearly communicated the message, "I want to talk."

That much "said," Joyce let out a hollow, low-pitched sound to signal her daughter in the kitchen to bring her computerized communication board to her. Amy moved quickly to do her mother's request, for Joyce enjoyed one remarkable physical boon: Using the two fingers over which she retained some slight control, she could actually type out a few words on her "com board." It was slow going, but effective.

With practiced skill, Amy positioned the board comfortably for her mom. Then she graciously bowed out of our company to give us privacy. We didn't need to worry about any part of our visit being overheard.

Alone again with Joyce, I was ready to listen. Rarely are our patients as eager as Joyce had been for an opportunity to talk about painful issues. Even her ravaged body conveyed a "let's get down to business" attitude. There would be no small talk between us.

"Joyce," I began, "I'm glad you asked me to come. What is it you'd like to talk about?"

An intense struggle to express herself ensued. Letter by letter, click by click, Joyce spelled out a deep cry of anguish: "I don't want to die, and there is nothing I can do about it!"

We sat in a long, sacred moment of silence. There was no gap to fill; I simply held her hand and waited. Joyce understood that we could have this difficult conversation, and that we would take whatever time was necessary for her to express her feelings.

I was aware that she probably had not risked being this nakedly vulnerable before. Oftentimes when patients try to talk with family about their deep fears and sadness, they are shut down, told to not give up hope, stay positive, and so forth.

Yet many dying patients long to have an open conversation, to express what this experience of dying is like for them, and how much they wrestle with their heavy feelings. Many who are terminally ill also need opportunities to protest out loud, "This isn't fair!"

My hope going into this visit was that Joyce could unburden herself. "What else do you want me to know about how you're feeling?"

Once again Joyce went straight to the heart of things, tapping with her workable index finger. Click, click, click. "I don't want to die." She paused to gather her strength. With great effort, she added, "BUT AT LEAST I CAN BE HOME WHEN MY GRANDKIDS COME, NOT GONE AT WORK LIKE BEFORE." A huge smile lit up her face as she tapped out the word *grandkids*.

"Yes, that's a very good thing!" I agreed, joining her husky laugh. We went on to talk about those kids she adored. She tapped out stories of their antics, of their sweetness when they crawled up beside her to snuggle. She shared their simple but profound questions about her disease and her suffering. "Grandma, what's wrong with your lap?" "Why can't you play on the floor with us?" "I want you to wrestle with me again."

Later, alone in the sanctuary of my car, I reflected on our encounter, as I do after each home visit. Joyce's words had struck me deeply. "At least I can be home when my grandkids come." She was facing an untimely and unfair death, and still was able to find something to be grateful for. "At least …"

Pulling into the office parking lot, I was feeling ashamed of my morning gripes. Spilled coffee? Tight shoes? While I wondered how to find time to catch up to myself, with each new dawn Joyce had to face giving up yet another piece of her life.

I sat there and cried.

During the next six months of visits preceding Joyce's death, the words *at least* became the signature of each conversation. She regularly wove them into her moment-by-moment reality, even as she struggled to come to terms with her impending death. "At least I can still lie in bed beside my husband at night." "Even if I can't eat at least I can taste things on my tongue." "At least all my children live close enough to stay with me." "At least my hair is washed today."

With each visit, I routinely read in Joyce's methodical communication her abiding gratitude for even the smallest things. She kept her sense of humor always, and I came to relish those moments when we could laugh together.

My last visit with Joyce stands out as the most memorable. Her husband had contacted me to report that she seemed especially emotional the past few days. Carl sensed the end was near, and would I please come? He sounded overwhelmed, and it was clear he needed some support himself. After all these months of patiently, lovingly listening to Joyce and caring for her every need, he was truly going to lose her! Faced with the inevitable, the burden of his own helplessness weighed heavily on him.

With conviction, I expressed my deep admiration for the dedicated care Carl had given Joyce all along, as well as my confidence that he was capable of hanging in there for her.

I reminded him how well he had managed so far, and how much his wife appreciated him.

Carl knew this was all true, and he seemed to find some consolation in the reassuring words, "at least" enough to return to Joyce's side.

When I arrived for our final visit, Joyce could not lift her head at all or control the drool escaping the side of her mouth. Her eyes, milky gray instead of blue, struggled to focus. Her bright, lime-colored loungewear belied her ravaged condition. And yet, she retained the barest ability to type with her index finger. It was still possible for us to "talk" about whatever could be said using the fewest words possible.

Joyce worked painfully at her board. "No time lft," she tapped out. "I so sad. No out." And then her shoulders shook as the sobs came without warning. She poured out her anguish, tears flowing, nose running, and drool making a slow stream down her chin onto a dish-towel bib. Again her finger tapped out a soul-wrenching message: "sposed to acpt it, jst cnt."

At that moment, it wasn't about how to respond—there was no good response. All I could do was bear witness in silence.

And then Joyce typed the very last words she would ever communicate to me. "At lst I can stl cry. ALS cnt take awy my trs."

This remains the most profound statement of gratitude I've ever encountered, and it has become a beacon for me. When I'm engulfed by the endless little trials and inconveniences of everyday life, tempted to wallow in self-pity, Joyce's face comes to mind. Her example shines brightly to guide my thoughts in a different direction.

I can tell you: Finding a way to be grateful and expressing it unclutters my heart and makes room for joy. Sometimes I can even be heard to say, "Thing are bad now, but at least we have time to make them better!"

BEFORE YOU GO

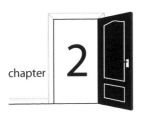

Lily

Advice from a Purple Poodle

Somehow, the act of self-giving is a personal power-releasing factor.

Dr. Norman Vincent Peale

Needless to say, it's easy enough to be generous and caring when we're happy, resources are plentiful, and it's all good. During those times I'm glad to pick up the dinner check, give extra time to a project, be that shoulder to cry on. But when I'm pressed by my busy agenda, and the debits of life seem to outnumber the credits, I can find myself pulling away, retreating to safe places.

When I began my work in hospice in 2006, there was so much to learn that my head hurt from cramming in new information. The job required me to travel constantly about the city—itself a tiring adjustment. Plus, there was an anxious gap between my last paycheck and the next, so money was tight. I was definitely running on empty.

During this time, I remember, a dear friend was experiencing her own hardships. Despite wanting to help, I felt constrained to measure out my time, possessions, and energy sparingly. Even digging deep, I could find barely enough strength to send her a heartfelt email.

I'm only human, of course. And yet I've encountered a few among us who seem able to give beyond ordinary capacity. They deliver just what's needed, at exactly the right moment. Sometimes these individuals aren't who you expect them to be. Lily, the 7-year-old daughter of one of our patients, was such a one.

You could see in one glance that Lily was an over-the-top girlie-girl, a pink-and-blonde dynamo in matching princess accessories. She was also the indulgent keeper of sundry stuffed animals about whom she was prone to burble torrents of chatter. The first thing she told me when we met was that we'd better be quiet because her "anmals" were taking their nap.

"Everybody's sleeping 'cept Emmie," she said, holding up a well-loved, stuffed purple poodle. (And why not a purple poodle, not a brown or white one, as befits a pink-thinking princess?) "'Cause she's gotta help me bake a cake."

"Hello, Miss Emmie," I said, smiling and patting her paw.

"You kin kiss her nose. She likes that."

And so I did, the first time I'd ever kissed a purple poodle. Besides making friends with Lily and Emmie, I enjoyed meeting the rest of the Terrell family as well—two charming young parents, Raquel and Frank. It was easy to see where Lily came by her bright and breezy ways.

Our reason for working with the Terrells for the past six months was not a happy one, however. Raquel Terrell, only 38 years old, was dying from a breast cancer that had metastasized throughout her body. Until the disease struck her down, Lily's young mom had been teaching French in a local high school and enjoying a full life with her family.

When we first met them, Raquel and Frank told us their special story, how Raquel had grown up in France but met Frank while visiting the United States. According to Frank, their first date was supposed to be a get-together for morning coffee but turned into an all-day event. They fell in love and married within a few months. Lily arrived two years later.

When Raquel and Frank had called hospice into their lives six months earlier, Raquel said her goal was to stay at home as long as possible. She hoped to share many precious moments with her family right beside her during her final days. But as her death drew closer, she changed her mind.

Now she fervently desired to spend her last moments in our inpatient unit (IPU). She told us why, very directly: "I want most to shield Frank and Lily from the image of my lifeless body here in the same bed that's been the center of our family life."

This made sense to her, so it made sense to us.

As the disease progressed, Raquel experienced extreme pain. Our medical directors and nursing staff were challenged to find ways to manage it well while Raquel remained at home. Still, she bravely determined to stay a while longer so that Lily could flutter in and out of her mom's room whenever she pleased. Sometimes she'd stop by just to watch Raquel lie quietly in her bed. Other times, Lily would climb up and sit beside her mom to read a book.

During one of my visits, Lily pranced into Raquel's room wearing her full princess regalia, including pink tulle tutu and oversized rhinestone tiara. Finding me there, she chirped, "Hi, Cherí! I came in to show mom my new dance. Wanna see?"

"I'd love to see your new dance," said I to the fairy princess.

"Me, too," Raquel said, laughing.

Lily twirled round and round at the foot of the bed, somehow balancing the tiara on her head. Suddenly she jumped to Raquel's side. "Mom," she mused with furrowed brow, "why can't I wear my sparkly flip-flops to school?"

"Because, *ma chèrie,* your feet will be so cold. The snow will fall on them."

"Oh." And off she went again.

Each time I visited Raquel, Lily would soon appear, chattering about her "anmals" and their antics, how Emmie had been sick, "but I made her all better," how Big Teddy was very naughty today. "He wouldn't take his nap!" Always she had to show me her newest girlie-girl flourish—be it glitter nail polish, pink lip gloss, or Jonas Brothers T-shirt. More than once I came home with newly painted pink fingernails.

🐾 🐾 🐾

Weeks passed, and Raquel's condition deteriorated. When the hospice nurse paid her early-morning visit, she noted signs that Raquel's death was imminent. She was barely responsive now, and her pain could no longer be managed successfully at home.

With Raquel's consent and Frank's support, hospice made the necessary arrangements to have her transported by ambulance to our inpatient facility. During the next week in the IPU, family and friends gathered by her side to say their good-byes. Most of the time, Lily was present and taking it all in—the tears, the laughter, even the moments when her mom cried out in pain.

One minute Lily would be focused intently on whatever was happening with her mom, and the next she'd be lost in some diversion. Her on-again, off-again engagement with the situation was typical behavior for a child coping with a dying parent. At one point she lay on her tummy on the floor, pretending to be swimming—perhaps truly swimming away from the sad reality of the moment. In her own way, she was slowly absorbing what dying meant.

During the last hours of Raquel's life, Lily was invited to choose one special teddy from among the many orphan bears who filled the cupboards at the nurse's station. Brand new, donated teddy bears are a key part of the comfort program at many hospices. Stuffed animals make soothing friends for children struggling to cope with grief and loss.

Lily chose a plush white teddy with big brown eyes and a soft smile. She named him Snowball and clung to him all the while she was in the room with her mom.

That entire day, Frank, Lily, Snowball, and a few other family members kept a tender watch over Raquel. Eventually, seeing that she was free of pain and sleeping deeply, they decided it was a good time to take a break and go to a nearby restaurant for dinner.

While her family sat wearily at the restaurant, raising a toast in her honor, Raquel quietly slipped away.

Raquel's timing illustrates a moving truth: Patients often die when their loved ones, who might have been sitting vigil for days, finally pull themselves away for a much-needed break. Did she somehow, at some level, arrange to spare her beloved family the heartache of watching her take her last breath? I believe so.

Shortly after Raquel's death, Frank requested that I make a home visit to talk with Lily. As I stepped into the Terrell's living room, she bounded toward me for a hug, her usual greeting.

"Lily—hello, sweetheart! So nice to see you!" I said, scooping her up. "Tell me, what's been going on with you? How are Emmie and Big Teddy and all your animals?"

"Good. But they fight sometimes. Daddy said I could only take one anmal to church, and I took LuLuBelle" (a one-eyed bunny). Before long, Lily was chattering about her mom's funeral, her cousins, the strange goings on. "I didn't like all the talking at church," she said, scrunching up her face. "But the food was yummy! I liked the brownies the best!"

Suddenly her face lit up. "Wait here—I'll be right back!" She was off in a flash, to return a few minutes later holding a velveteen pink dress with puff sleeves. "See what I wore to mom's special day?"

"Isn't that just beautiful, Lily!"

"An' did you know my cousin Marcie was there? She tol' me her mom was sick, too." Her eyes lit up again. "Wait—I wanna show you my new teddy bear. I picked him out myself!"

Off she went and returned hugging Snowball to her chest. "See?" she said, tenderly smoothing his scruffy white fur. Then her brow furrowed. "Hey, where do your nurses get all those teddys? And how come you give 'em to kids?"

"Well, Lily, kind people give them to us," I told her. "They want kids to have a special friend to hold when they feel scared or sad, or miss their mom."

"I miss my mom," Lily said in a small voice.

I nodded. "I know you miss your mom, sweetheart. The nurses know, too. Kids want to keep the person they love with them always, and they miss them so much when they're gone."

As Lily pondered this, her face brightened. "Do you know any more kids with a mom that died?"

"Yes, I do—I know lots of kids with a mom or dad that died," I said, wanting to reassure her she wasn't alone. Children in Lily's situation can feel isolated, or even believe no one else ever had a parent die, just because nobody told them otherwise.

Lily paused to absorb my response. Then she spun around and ran to her bedroom, calling "I'll be right back!" A closet door squeaked, followed by scuffling noises. I could just pick up the muffled sound of items softly hitting the floor.

A few moments later, she appeared and gleefully presented me with her cherished purple poodle! "Here, Cherí. I want you to give Emmie to another little girl who doesn't have a mom anymore."

I was stunned. "Oh, but Lily, you love Emmie so much! Are you sure you want to give her away?"

She nodded emphatically. "I want to—you know—what do you call it when people give you teddy bears?"

"Donate?"

"Yeah! I want to donate my poodle to a girl who's sad 'cause her mom's dying." She seemed captured by the idea.

With Frank's permission, I accepted Lily's humble donation. Frank, too, was deeply touched by his young daughter's pure generosity. This was an amazing little girl! After all, barely two weeks had passed since her own mother's death.

"Thank you so much, Lily," I said. "You're a special girl to give away something you love so much!"

Today Lily's purple poodle occupies a prominent position on my office bookshelf to commemorate her charitable spirit. ("House rules," of course, disallowed my passing Emmie along for hygienic reasons.) Instead, she's become my marker for selfless giving—a simple reminder that living with generosity during our hardest moments may be key to helping ourselves keep things in perspective.

BEFORE YOU GO

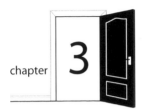

Mary

Holding On ... And Letting Go

No matter what one endures ... the imperative to affirm one's power persists, even in those encased in the sickest, most ghostly bodies.

Roxana Badine

In hospice work, one of the most common questions family members pose to staff is as succinct—and profound—as it gets: How long does my loved one have to live?

As medical professionals, we hesitate to give an answer because we're often proved wrong. Staff are amazed by the patient whose will to live sustains him or her far beyond what we would ever have predicted. Individuals who have gone without nourishment for days, whose condition has drastically declined, who seemed at death's door, somehow hang on—sometimes in order to see a loved one for the last time.

There is indeed something awesome about that will to affirm life at all costs.

It's a truism in hospice that—usually—"people die the way they lived." Another way to put it, based on what I've seen, is that people often draw on the same attitudes and coping skills they used during life to face their dying. Most surrender to the inevitable as they can, in stages. Some can let go with a measure of graciousness. Others cannot.

Unsurprisingly, those individuals notable in life for a certain stubbornness or unbending nature will refuse to be "gathered" at all into the night.

Never have I witnessed a more convincing demonstration of this last stance than with our patient Mary, a 67-year-old woman dying of advanced cervical cancer. Mary had been in hospice home care for only eight weeks. Her 20-something granddaughter, Elise, had been her primary caregiver since Mary's terminal diagnosis a year ago. Elise worked as a waitress to support the two of them in a small, one-bedroom apartment.

This little family had its share of mystery. Mary's own daughter was nowhere to be found, her history unknown. The merest notation in the caseworker's file attested to her existence. Evidently she had abandoned Elise early on.

Once Mary had been Elise's caretaker; now the roles were reversed, with perhaps the same level of desperation on young Elise's part. The team knew that Mary would soon be unresponsive and unable to make decisions about her own care. To ensure she would receive the kind of treatment she wanted at the last, it was vital we obtain a Power of Attorney for Health Care, or POAHC.

In many states the POAHC is preferred over a Living Will because it specifically designates a legal representative (usually a family member) to make and enforce health care decisions on behalf of the patient, whereas a Living Will only states the wishes of the patient. Thus, a POAHC often makes it easier for the family to make end-of-life decisions.

We were making a second home visit to inform Mary of her options.

It was early afternoon on a cool, breezy September day

when our party of three—nurse, social worker, and I—stepped into Elise and Mary's claustrophobic world. A hospital bed dominated the modest living room so that it seemed to pull the bare, white walls in close around its occupant, a frail, small woman dressed in bright pink pajamas. Someone had chosen that wonderful color with care, I thought.

Although Mary seemed to catch sight of us with a sideways glance, she didn't acknowledge our presence in any way. She only sat up in the bed, her legs hung over the side, her tiny frame slightly bent—just enough for her to lean over and rest her elbows on the bedside table. She kept her head bent low, so we couldn't quite see her face.

For all of us, it was a discomforting sight, but we had to respect Mary's choice to sit up. I slowly approached her bedside and bent down to speak to her. "What pretty pink pajamas! They match the blanket on your bed."

Mary only groaned loudly.

At this, our nurse Carol stepped immediately to her side and asked, "Are you in pain?"

Again Mary groaned.

"Maybe you should lie down," Carol said gently, reaching to help her lie back.

"No, thank you," Mary mumbled. At least she was communicating with us, even if she refused to accede to her own comfort.

Carol threw me a look that said, *Uh-oh, this could be a tough one.* We knew Mary's sitting had to be putting more pressure on her abdomen, which could only aggravate her pain. Despite this, she persisted in her contrary posture, head bowed low and face hidden.

"Are you sure you wouldn't like to lie down for a while?" Carol asked softly. "I can help you stretch out and be more comfortable."

"No, thank you."

"She sits up *all* the time," Elise noted, shaking her head with exasperation. "I can't even hardly get her to lay down for a minute to go to sleep. She so stubborn, it's c-r-a-z-y, and she drivin' *me* crazy!"

Mary sat unmoved. Only once, when the social worker explained the Power of Attorney document, did she slowly lift her head to nod that she understood. She showed us a haggard face but one with jaw set, as she grasped the pen and signed the document. Then she dropped her head down as before.

If Mary wouldn't lie down, we thought, perhaps she'd let us prop her up with the myriad pillows strewn about the bed. Several times we solicited her cooperation in this simple compromise measure, but she would not—or *could* not—relax her guard.

Elise was beyond frustrated. Throwing up her hands, she declared, "My grandma thinks if she lies down she's gonna die, and Lord knows she's not gonna let that happen!" Clearly she wanted Mary to *please, please, just lie back!*

It was hard on all of us to stand by helplessly, but there was nothing else to be done for Mary without her consent. We quietly took our leave, apparently unnoticed by our patient.

When the team met to review Mary's status later that week, her campaign to sit upright came under discussion. We were confident that as her condition worsened, Mary herself would seek to relieve her discomfort and finally lie down. For now, we agreed, her need to exercise some power over her condition seemed paramount. Regardless, we would defer to her choice in the matter.

By the time I made my last home visit a month later, Mary's condition had deteriorated to the point that she was no longer verbal in any way. According to Elise, she was barely taking in any fluids and had stopped eating altogether. This development was not surprising. It showed a typical downward progression that we'd seen many times before in cancer patients.

Through it all, Mary remained unbending. I arrived to find her sitting upright in exactly the same posture as before—elbows leaning on her bedside table, head bowed. Her tiny frame, so diminished by weight loss, was drowning in a yellow print housedress several sizes too big. Flowery sleeves puddled over onto the bedside table as if they were extensions of her body. Matching yellow slippers hung loosely from her feet, just barely holding on.

Approaching her bed, I leaned gently toward her. "Hello, Mary. Here you are, holding on so bravely." Unable to speak or lift her head, Mary could not have mumbled a response even if she'd wanted to—which, I'm sure, she did not.

Yet this visit was a special occasion. Two of Mary's sisters, Ella and Doris, had traveled all the way from their homes in Mississippi to be with her.

For me, it was both an unexpected pleasure and a relief to meet these two full-figured, soft-spoken women. Ella and Doris hugged me warmly and thanked me for being there to help. It was good to know Mary and Elise would have some solid family support during this tough time.

When we sat down together at the kitchen table, there was deep concern for Mary's situation, but relaxed talk and laughter, too. The room itself seemed to expand and breathe a little easier with their presence. Little by little, I learned something of Mary's story. According to Ella and Doris, she had been a stubborn one from the beginning.

"Way back, Mary moved up here all by herself, away from the rest of us," Doris recounted. "You know, she was gonna live how *she* saw fit. But she did it, she made it okay." She chuckled under her breath. "She so bullheaded but she done proved she could do it."

Over the years, the family in Mississippi hadn't heard much from their long-lost sheep. "How did you feel about Mary living so far away all these years?" I wondered aloud.

"Oh, we missed our sister," Ella said.

"We wished we lived closer," Doris agreed. "It's hard to see her so miserable. She believe if she lay down, she'll die. Every time we try 'n lay her down, she jus' make a fuss. So we leave her be."

"Well, it gotta hurt her to do it but she keep doin' it," Ella added in a tone of resignation. "When we was kids Mary was always tryin' to be the boss over everybody. She never listened to nobody then and she ain't listenin' now."

Despite myself, strains of *Mary, Mary, quite contrary* played in the back of my mind. Still, along with her sisters, I had to give Mary my grudging admiration. She was determined to die as she saw fit.

Dr. Ernest Rosenbaum, a noted oncologist and author, has observed the attitudes of many terminal cancer patients. He posits that those who assume an aggressive fighting posture against their disease strengthen their will to live. Mary was giving us a literal demonstration.

༄ ༄ ༄

Some three days later, in the early morning hours, our 24/7 team received a tearful call from Elise. Moments ago, at 3 a.m., she'd gotten up to check on her grandma and found her dead. Mary had died sitting up, with elbows resting on the bedside table!

The hospice nurse who pronounced the death wanted to allow Elise some private time with her grandma before calling for the funeral staff to step in. Typically the nurse bathes and clothes the body, then positions the loved one for family to attend in peace for a while. But Mary's insistence on sitting up, right to the end, presented a unique challenge: The nurse had to coax and massage her body into a reclining position.

Thanks to these ministrations, however, Mary finally lay back peacefully with eyes closed and hands folded gently over her pink blanket. Elise was greatly comforted at the sight of her grandma completely at rest. This was the way to bid farewell.

When we reviewed Mary's case at the next team meeting, we all marveled at her tenacity. Rarely had we witnessed such a force of will coming from one so frail. Had it been her fears that kept her sitting up? Did she ever express affection or longing for anyone? What had been her hopes? Dreams? Regrets?

We didn't have the answers. But with her iron will to sit into eternity, Mary seemed to model the attitude of a textbook "survivor"—someone conditioned by early adversity or hardship to perceive threats everywhere. Someone bound to bear down and *endure* when she could neither fight nor flee such threats. Such a one can never relax her guard, lest she be defeated.

Thus Mary's stance could be seen as the last act of a woman determined to allow herself no quarter or comfort, never mind the others in her world. There are those moments in life when, having done what we could, exhaling into a gentle surrender seems much the wiser choice than clenching our teeth and refusing to bend. But how and when do we arrive at that point of acceptance?

It's precisely *there*, at that tipping point, that hospice is poised to assist patients. It might be a powerful word of pastoral counseling … a forgiving message from someone long ago dismissed from our lives … a last touch from a loved one or caregiver sitting by. Or simple pain relief.

Even, it seems, it could be taking a little time to write down (or dictate to another) what we think our lives have been about. As this book goes to press, a form of legacy writing known as dignity therapy is gaining favor in hospices around the world.

Dignity therapy involves asking an individual with a terminal condition questions about their life history, their values and motivations, and their work. The goal is to help them think about what they want their final legacy to be. What is it they want to leave for the next generation?

The individual is then helped to craft a concrete document or transcription that can be passed down.

By all indications, the process is highly effective in helping individuals come to see their life and death in a new light—finding in them a deeper meaning and purpose. Sharing a life story can also bring improved communication, or even reconciliation, with family members. At the very least, patients have the comfort of knowing their words will transcend their death.

It's tempting to wonder how such a process might have impacted Mary or Elise, or Mary's family back in Mississippi—or possibly even her long-estranged daughter. Even a legacy document that's discovered long after its author's death can bring healing in unforeseen ways.

According to Harvey Max Chochinov, a psychiatrist researching the effects of dignity therapy on quality of life, individuals use the process for a wide array of purposes, from apologizing for squandered gifts or opportunities, to recording the derivation of a daughter's name or other obscure biographical information.

We'll never know how things might have played out differently in Mary's case. But like her, we're all destined to struggle in the balance between holding on and letting go. Between resisting and finally accepting *what is*.

In this struggle, we have available to us at least one tried and true way to access the soul-soothing power of surrender:

the world-famous Serenity Prayer of Alcoholics Anonymous: *God, grant me the serenity to accept the things I cannot change, courage to change the things I can, and wisdom to know the difference.*"

Sadly, it seems Mary died with little serenity.

BEFORE YOU GO

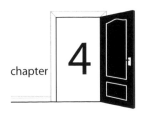

chapter 4

Harold

Don't Wait, Open Your Gifts

Waiting for the fish to bite
or waiting for wind to fly a kite.
Or waiting around for Friday night ...
Everyone is just waiting.

Dr. Seuss

It was an unusually hot day in early June when I accompanied Carrie and Kristin, our hospice social worker and nurse case manager, to the new patient's home. Harold was an elderly man whose heart was failing. In fact, he had less than six months to live. He knew what to expect from our hospice team—his wife, Martha, had died six years ago from complications of cancer, passing away peacefully on our inpatient unit. Now Harold wanted hospice to pay him a visit.

We parked our cars on the street and walked up the driveway, noting the grungy Christmas wreath and lights that hung forlornly above the garage door. It was common for frail elderly people to avoid taking down seasonal decorations.

We weren't surprised, either, when a large and dusty artificial Christmas tree greeted us upon entering the house. A couple of brown oak leaves, probably blown in from outside, clung to a cobweb woven among the tree's branches. A few dull ornaments were sparsely hung among the burnt-out white twinkle lights.

Most poignant of all, an array of faded red- and green-wrapped gifts, their bows intact, lay unopened under the tree. Each had its gift tag, and I could read *To: Harold, From: Martha* identifying the gift nearest to me.

Carrie and I exchanged a glance but said nothing. Instead we took a few minutes to admire the many smiling photos of Harold, Martha, and their family scattered around the room—on the piano, knick-knack shelves, and end tables.

Harold and Martha looked to be a picture-perfect "Ozzie and Harriet" couple, straight out of the 1950s. In each Sunday-best portrait, Martha wore an embroidered or polka-dot shirtwaist dress, matching pumps, and "church hat." Harold, standing alongside her in suit and tie, beamed proudly. His hair was neatly combed, Bryl-creemed, and precisely parted on the right.

But Martha was gone six years now, and today we found Harold lying quietly in his recliner, wearing only a plain white undershirt and Wrangler blue jeans. His hair was unkempt.

I smiled hello. "Those are wonderful family photos, Harold! You must miss your wife very much." Kristin chimed in to note how well the family had coordinated with hospice to take care of Martha during her last days, and to recap how things had gone since.

"How are you feeling today?" she began her assessment. "Is your pain manageable?" When she finished, we worked with Harold to set the stage for the ongoing care he wanted. We also addressed, one by one, the big emotional issues of the moment: Have you had a chance to talk with everyone in your family? Is there anyone else you'd like us to contact? Are your affairs arranged the way you want them?

Harold did his best to respond to our comments and queries, smiling and nodding here and there, though he drew his breath with difficulty. By the time our visit drew to a close, we felt we'd covered all the bases. Things had gone well.

Several weeks passed. Our warm Wisconsin June had morphed into a scorching July. After repeated home visits with Harold, he'd grown to trust me enough to share some of his best hopes and memories. He especially enjoyed reminiscing on topics of faith and family. Harold was a man with a long-standing belief in God and a deep conviction that he'd be with Martha in heaven soon.

During this visit, we were joined by Harold's son Darrell, his dad's primary caregiver. With all of us sitting down together, maybe this was the right moment to prompt, "Well, Harold, are you going to have Christmas soon? There sure are a lot of presents under that tree!"

Harold made no reply, but Darrell protested immediately. "No! Those have been there since my mother died!"

Wow. I was a little surprised that Darrell had answered so quickly for his dad. "So is that how you feel too, Harold?"

"Yeah. I guess we just never got around to opening 'em," he mumbled, and then added, as if this were the obvious explanation, "Martha picked 'em out just a few weeks before she died." No matter that the tree and gifts remained untouched for six years, the two of them clearly wanted the scene left undisturbed.

So be it.

In hospice, a key part of assessing new patients is to inquire as sensitively as possible about any losses they might be contending with, past or present. As grief counselors, we believe it's essential that patients be given all the opportunity they need to unburden themselves.

Again and again we've seen that lending a listening ear

and caring presence can facilitate deep emotional release and healing. Some patients talk with ease and openly share their painful emotions, fears, and worries. Others do not.

Whichever way they lean, we consider it a great gift to follow their lead. In Harold's case, like many in his generation, he was simply unable, or unwilling, to articulate his deepest thoughts and feelings. Even after coming to trust me, he declined to share how he felt about living without Martha all these years, or how he felt about his own illness and approaching death.

I felt bound to respect his silence.

As expected, Harold's heart disease progressed rapidly. Like Martha, he elected to spend his last days on our inpatient unit rather than at home. During that four-week period, we paid careful attention to every detail of his comfort care, including, of course, making sure his hair was clean and precisely parted on the right side.

All the while, his unopened gifts lay gathering dust under the tree at home. Harold would never know what Martha had chosen just for him. Although he never said so, I suspect Harold believed it would be dishonoring to Martha to enjoy her gifts without her there. Maybe preserving them intact was his way of keeping her memory whole and alive, and not upsetting Darrell.

Unlike Harold, many of our terminally ill patients do choose to affirm whatever life they have remaining *now*, this very moment. They are strongly motivated to make the most of any hidden blessings. Given a last chance, they'll open that box of chocolates. They seize the day and grab the opportunity to go places they always wanted to go. They savor even the smallest of gifts along the way.

As Dr. Ira Byock, the renowned expert in palliative medicine, notes in his book, *The Four Things That Matter Most*, such patients often find the courage to say the truly important things: I love you. I forgive you. Please forgive me. Thank you.

Harold had his reasons for making the choices he did. While I confess that a very human part of me wanted to "fix things"—to nudge him into the present moment where he could enjoy his gifts from Martha—I knew it was his call to make, not mine.

Still, the image of those dust-covered presents scattered around the spindly trunk of a dingy artificial Christmas tree has stayed with me, a sad symbol of years not fully lived, and happiness shortchanged. Was I living my own life to the full? What gifts, talents, and invitations to adventure had *I* left unexplored or unappreciated?

Plenty. What came to mind first was a bit of a revelation. Once upon a time I sang solos in church services and even participated in local musical productions. Why did I set all that aside? It's been so long since I felt that special joy of singing with my whole being.

Other gifts of opportunity I managed to overlook. Why didn't I go visit friends and family living abroad when I had the chance? I could have visited Europe at virtually no expense. For that matter, I wish I'd flown out to California and surprised my folks on their special anniversary.

Was I really *that* busy?

And why haven't I taken those cooking classes ... reconnected with that old friend ... planted a rose garden ... read one new best-seller ... walked more with my husband ... whiled away an afternoon doing *nothing*? I started paying attention to the all the little stuff that was really big stuff.

I took note of the unsolicited blessings sprinkled like glitter over my everyday life, such as the simple kindness of strangers—the driver who waved me into line ahead of him during rush-hour traffic that morning, the saleswoman at the Stop-N-Go who kept her smile when I tipped over the display of key chains at her cash register.

Whose life hasn't been touched by such small gestures?

On the other end of the spectrum, some gifts I saw were lavish gifts that poured over my life in perfect fulfillment of my heart's desire—for one, my son Derek, conceived and born after years of struggling to become pregnant.

Other powerful gifts came disguised as hardship and adversity, or wrapped in sorrow and loss. Only with time and perspective have they revealed their worth in growth. I never had the four children I dreamed of, but I was able to go to graduate school and find a career I love.

Whose life hasn't had similar twists and turns? You get the point.

These days, I accept the gifts as they come to me. I look for, acknowledge, and take action on those things I've been blessed with. The inner drive to "Just do it!" pushes me to reach toward all life has to offer. Like a child on Christmas morning, I search out every last gift still waiting to be opened and let fly the wrappers and ribbon!

BEFORE YOU GO

BEFORE YOU GO

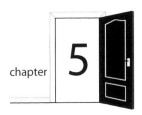

Shirley

BEFORE YOU GO

When Truth Can Shatter

Everything I have ever learned in my lifetime leads back to this: the fires and the black river of loss whose other side is salvation ...

Mary Oliver

We struggle to find any legitimate way to avoid telling those we love the truth when it's going to break their hearts. Of course we do. Who wants to be the bearer of bad—very bad—news? We hesitate, procrastinate, protect. Even in the telling, we fight the temptation to somehow soften the blow.

When the truth means a new, life-shattering reality for children, resistance intensifies by a magnitude. Our staff dreaded this exact dilemma with the Kemp family. Thirty-six-year-old Shirley Kemp had been diagnosed nine months earlier with an aggressive form of uterine cancer that had proven unresponsive to treatment. The brutal fact was, she would die soon.

Naturally, Shirley and her husband Roger found themselves wanting to protect their children—Ashley, age 9, and Jared, age 6—from the truth. Shirley's raging cancer had taken no notice of what two children needed.

This fact added a crushing burden to Roger Kemp's already unbearable load. He was barely staggering through his days, literally suffocating under a blanket of doom.

Roger's anguish drew the concern of our hospice nurse, Kristin. During her second solo visit to the Kemp home, she took him aside and gently probed, "How are you holding up, Roger? Is there any way we can help you through this?"

Roger grabbed hold of the lifeline. Maybe he wasn't completely alone in the face of the disaster besetting his family. "How do we handle all this without the kids finding out their mom is going to die?" he blurted.

Kristin reflected silently for a long moment. She looked Roger in the eye and said evenly, "Maybe you might want to consider telling them the truth."

As Roger struggled to take this in, Kristin added in the same even tone, "Our grief counselor is very good in these situations. She'd be more than happy to talk with you and Shirley about how to help the children through all of this."

Roger wanted all the help he could get. On her way home, Kristen left me a voice message describing the dilemma of these two devoted parents immobilized by grief. "Cherí, they're in such turmoil, it's horrible to see. Please, would you call them and follow up?"

When Roger and I spoke by phone, he was desperate for some assurance that there was a way to help his children. What did the experts say? Did I have any experience with this situation?

"I'm open to whatever hospice recommends," he vowed.

Roger and I decided a home visit would be the best start. I could get acquainted with the family, especially Jared and Ashley. I needed to meet these two little people and get to know them. How did they feel about their mom being so sick? What was in their heart of hearts?

Besides which, I would need some time to build up my own courage. Although I had worked with children coping with the loss of a parent, I'd never been asked to help deliver such shattering news.

Until nine months ago, the Kemp family had lived a simple and happy life, content to live within their means. What they wanted most was to create a loving, secure home, and this they had done. The foursome occupied a small house in a tree-filled, middle-class neighborhood where Ashley and Jared walked the two blocks to school. Activities revolved around getting together with extended family nearby. Beyond that, Roger and Shirley's volunteer efforts at the children's elementary school kept them all busy.

Now we were about to detonate a nuclear bomb over their happy home.

After pulling into the Kemp driveway for my first visit, I sat for a moment. A light spring rain was falling, but my heart was as heavy as the overcast sky. Children need their mother! What a rotten break life was serving up to Ashley and Jared! It was so unfair. Shaking my head, I gathered my materials and started up the sidewalk.

Roger was standing sentinel at the front door, dressed in shorts and a T-shirt. As I approached, he joined me outside on the front step. A white metal awning shielded us from the rain. "Thanks for coming. I just wanted to meet you and tell you about the kids before you talk with them."

I smiled my greetings as we shook hands. "It's good to meet you in person, Roger. And, please, call me Cherí."

Roger led me into a small living room and invited me to sit down. He jumped right in: "Ashley's the oldest, she's very talkative but hasn't said a lot about how she feels since her mom got sick. She's always serious. Maybe she just doesn't want to cause us any extra worry. But she's really bossy with Jared. I'm guessing she thinks she's helping us by insisting he behave. Most of the time, though, Ashley and Jared get along pretty well."

He took a breath, then added, "Ashley does great in school—a straight *A* student. But she's almost too grown up."

"Does she stick close by her mom most of the time?"

"Oh, yeah." Roger said, blinking back tears. Almost whispering, he confided, "She's so much her mom's little girl. She'll be devastated when Shirley dies. That's why I don't want her to know the truth."

I nodded. "And how about Jared? How's he coping with everything?"

"Jared likes to be silly, always goofing around. A real chatterbox, too. It's almost like he doesn't care much that his mom's so sick, but I know he does. I'm afraid he won't know what to do when he finds out Shirley's dying. He's so young to have such serious information." Roger took a deep breath and concluded, "He shouldn't have to deal with this at his age."

My thoughts exactly.

Roger had described behavior typical of children in this situation. To a fair degree, we at hospice can predict how children will react to the news that their mom was going to die. None of which eased the burden of telling them the truth. Was it cruel to be kind? Or kind to be cruel?

Jared and Ashley sat waiting to meet me at the kitchen table.

"Hi, kids—I'm Cherí," I announced. "You must be Ashley," I said, turning first to the brown-haired ragamuffin regarding me warily. "I've heard lots about you from your dad."

Ashley looked a little surprised. But she gave me a shy hello, pushing a few strands of loose hair off her forehead. I couldn't help thinking that her dad must have dressed her in a rush this morning and forgotten to brush her hair.

"And you're Jared, right?" I said, turning to the sweaty-headed boy who sat fidgeting in his chair. "I hear you've got some good stories!"

Jared grinned.

"Kids, I'm here to help take care of your mom. You know, she's told me so many good things about you two. Your dad, too. I'm really glad I get to meet you."

Both youngsters smiled.

"You know, when a mommy or daddy is very sick, it can be a hard time for kids. So sometimes I help them do special stuff."

Ashley listened intently. Jared, intrigued, jumped up to peer inside my shopping bag of craft supplies.

"Is this the special stuff?"

"Yup. I brought a cool project for us to work on together, if you want."

Ashley and Jared looked on expectantly. Removing one item at a time, I laid out all the "special" bag contents on the table—balsa-wood box, poster paints, brushes, colored markers, glitter, scratch paper, plastic cups. Last of all, I pulled out a pad of yellow stationery bordered by colorful flowers.

I had their full attention. With deliberate care, I picked up the small, unpainted wooden box, turned it over appreciatively, and said, "This is what we call a memory box. You can decorate it with paint and anything else you like. Then when it dries, we can write down your favorite family memories and put them inside the box. So what do you think, guys?"

Ashley and Jared beamed their approval.

"So let's get our special project underway, shall we? Why don't you two decide who's going to decorate the sides, who'll paint the cover."

"I wanna paint the cover," Ashley cried instantly.

"Yeah—okay." Jared agreed easily. His big sister would do a better job with the cover—no argument! His job would be to paint the sides just right.

Things were going about as well as I could hope.

We got under way. Soon enough, Jared showed himself to be the sweet goof his dad had described, while Ashley seemed totally absorbed by her efforts.

Then Jared spoke up suddenly. "Yeah, it's hard my mom's sick. Did you know this summer I couldn't go camping with my dad 'cause he had to stay home 'n help Mom? Ashley didn't even *wanna* go."

I cocked my head toward Ashley as if to say, *Won't you tell us what you think, too?* But, no—not yet. In a flash, Jared picked up the story, "Ashley likes to stay here with mom and be in her room."

"Yeah, but it's not 'cause I don't like camping!" she squawked back. "I just didn't feel like going that time. I'll go next summer when Mom's better."

My heart wrenched at her words. "Lots of kids feel that way," I said.

Ashley went back to concentrating on her painting. The two of them took turns brushing on paint in repeated efforts to achieve perfection. In the end, Jared's contribution was a series of dynamic red and yellow splotches on the sides of the box. Ashley's final application of a vivid turquoise gave the finishing touch to their masterpiece.

"Beautiful job, Ashley and Jared!" Then, with pen and special stationery poised before me, I asked the big question. "So now, guys, what memories can you think of that I can write down?"

Both kids began to chatter about their favorite family times—Ashley giving the facts, and Jared adding the flare.

"Let's write down our trip to the waterpark!" Ashley sang out, her eyes lighting up.

"Yeah, let's do that one!" gushed Jared. "An' did you know they had cartoons all over the walls, only they didn't get the ninja guy right—he's not yellow, he's kinda green. An' did you know we couldn't get past the big ladder in the middle of the pool, 'n we had to get all the way around it to get to the …" And on and on.

The kids called up memories of their many happy visits to

their cousins, of summer camping trips, Christmas surprises, special birthdays.

My job was to transcribe these shiny-bright memories with the greatest of care onto individual sheets of stationery. When neither child could think of anything more to add, we ceremoniously folded each written remembrance. Then Ashley and Jared took turns placing each treasured memory in the box, one by one.

Appearing satisfied with the results, Ashley pushed her chair away from the table and declared, "I'm gonna go check on Mom." And off she went. With Ashley gone, Jared gave one last look of approval before announcing, "I'm gonna go play Ninja!"

When I showed Roger the memory box, he was pleased. He grasped immediately how powerful a symbol of remembrance he held in his hands. That such a solid token of Shirley's memory would be forever available to the children consoled him greatly. This little box, at least, would be indestructible!

Now was the moment to reassure him about his worst fears. "Roger, I think it's okay to tell Ashley and Jared what's going on," I began.

"You do?" Roger asked doubtfully.

"Yes, I do. They're both aware things have changed in your family. This much I can assure you. People who work with kids tell us that they sense—even deeply know—when something important is changing in their world. That's been my experience, too. But when kids don't get confirmation of what they already suspect, their worst fears can run wild."

Roger nodded sadly.

"If they're not told what to expect, Ashley and Jared will try to puzzle out the truth on their own. Instead of feeling safe and protected, they may feel anxious or even guilty—like they're somehow responsible."

It might have been my imagination but I thought Roger looked awfully pale. My heart went out to him. "You're right, Roger," I said, "this situation is so harsh. But just imagine how betrayed Ashley and Jared would feel if their mom vanished without a word of goodbye!

"You can't change the situation. But if you help them digest what's happening as things move along, they'll know they can trust you for the truth—and they'll find huge comfort in that."

Reluctantly, Roger agreed.

ఌ ఌ ఌ

The moment of truth had arrived. Our hospice team—nurse Kristin, social worker Julie, and I—converged on the Kemp's doorstep with heavy hearts. We had come to care about this family, and we would witness much heartbreak today.

Roger and Shirley had prepped Ashley and Jared for this meeting. They knew we were there to talk about their mom's sickness, and that we wanted them there, too, because they were so important to the family.

We all gathered in the living room. Shirley sat on the sofa, enfolded in a blanket, a royal blue scarf wrapped around her bald head. Despite the regal headdress, her face betrayed exhaustion. Jared, quiet and attentive, sat beside his mom. Roger sat down in his recliner, and Ashley soon folded herself on the floor at his feet.

We took our places on the extra chairs brought in from the kitchen and looked on silently as Kristin checked Shirley's vital signs and jotted down the numbers. Then she put aside her notebook and looked directly at the children. She cleared her throat and spoke calmly.

"Jared and Ashley, your mom and dad asked us to come today to help them have a big talk with you," she began. "You know your mom is so sick with cancer. All the doctors have tried very hard to help her. They wanted to stop the cancer with the right medicine."

The children listened, wide-eyed.

"Sometimes, for some people," Kristin went on, "the medicine works really well. But for other people, it doesn't work so well. For your mom, the medicine is not working. The doctors can't find any way to help her get better."

Kristin paused and nodded toward me.

"And so, Ashley and Jared," I said slowly, "Since the medicine isn't working, and the doctors don't have anything else they can try, the cancer has gotten much, much worse." My next words caught in the back of my throat. "We are so very sorry to tell you, this means your mom can't get better, and she is going to die."

The moment was excruciating. Ashley and Jared stared at me.

"She's not going to die today," I continued in the same slow manner. "In fact, she probably has many weeks to live. We don't know for sure."

Ashley looked stricken. Jared shot alarmed looks back and forth from one to the other of us. *Steady, steady*, I thought, my heart pounding. "We know this must be so hard to understand." With that, I turned to Roger and Shirley and asked quietly, "Do either of you want to say anything?"

Shirley gently shook her head no. Roger slid to the edge of his chair and spoke softly. "Kids, your mom and I don't want you to be afraid. These ladies are here to help us with all of this stuff. You know we both love you and wish we didn't have to tell you this bad news."

Silence filled the room.

"Ashley, Jared, do you have any questions?" I asked. "Because usually there are lots of questions that kids ask."

Ashley locked eyes with her dad and implored, "Will my mom be here for my birthday?"

Words failed Roger, and he turned to Kristin for help. "Probably not, Ashley," she responded softly. "Your birthday is almost a year away, and the doctors don't think your mom will live that long." She stopped for a moment. "I'm really so sorry about that, sweetheart."

As if it all suddenly made sense to her, Ashley stood up, facing her dad. "So Mom is going to die?"

"Yes." Roger's voice was barely audible. Ashley collapsed onto his lap, sobbing. Roger cradled her wordlessly while Jared looked on, frozen.

It was agony.

After another long moment, Shirley moved closer to Jared and, leaning into him, put her hand on his. To everyone's surprise, she seemed to have drawn a spark of energy from the moment, enough to address her children in a calm, steady voice:

"Ashley and Jared, this is terrible, I know. But for now I'm feeling pretty good. I'm strong enough to be awake sometimes during the day. We can still have fun playing games together." Her voice remained calm. "Your dad is here, and he'll always be here for you. We don't have to think about my dying right now. We can think about how I should live and what special things we can still do together. Okay?"

"But why did you tell us?" Jared demanded.

"Because we want you to have time to ask questions like this," Roger answered. "And we don't want you to have a terrible surprise when it happens."

All was silence except for the muffled sound of Ashley crying.

"Do either of you have any more questions?" I asked finally. Ashley and Jared glared glumly in our direction and shook their heads. Again we assured them we would answer any questions they had. "We understand you don't want to ask us anything right now. But that might change. If it does, you can ask us anything you want, okay?"

It was time to leave the family alone. We conferred a moment with Roger and Shirley, scheduled our next visit, and left. Outside the three of us hugged wordlessly and returned to our cars.

❦ ❦ ❦

As awful as the moment of reckoning had been, over the next several weeks, we witnessed something remarkable. As Shirley slowly grew worse, the children's openness with her increased proportionately. There were moments of tears and sadness. But there were also moments of joy. The family basked often in the glow of gestures both children repeatedly made toward their mother. They expressed their great love for her in both words and acts.

The whole family took time for extra bedtime hugs and kisses. They read special stories together. They made more happy memories.

During one home visit, I found all four Kemps gathered around a photo album. Shirley and Roger were laughing and teasing Ashley and Jared about their baby pictures. "Remember how we called you Baby J?" "Look how tiny you were, Ashley!" The delight was palpable as they shared the private memories and catchphrases that made them a family.

Our reward for going the distance with the Kemps was to see how much they grew in their ability to share openly what everyone was seeing and feeling. The children asked many questions as they came up, and either we or their parents were there to answer them.

On one occasion Ashley wanted to know if her mom would be buried in the ground. When told yes, Jared chimed in, "We should get mom a blue casket—it's her favorite color." This led to a forthright conversation about why we have the funeral rituals that we do.

What's more, the Kemp children were able to enjoy another whole dimension of support. They now had many opportunities to talk with their teachers and schoolmates about what was happening at home. Parents of their classmates rallied around the family, fixed meals, babysat, and doled out extra measures of love and kindness to Ashley and Jared.

Not a day would pass without someone making a helping gesture toward the Kemp family. They found themselves buoyed by this sea of tenderness and generosity. Ashley and Jared witnessed firsthand the power of a community reaching out to help and comfort its own.

Would the Kemp family have opened to such an intimate sense of community without the storm of truth breaking over them? Perhaps, in the end, Ashley and Jared were as blessed by knowing the truth as they were scorched by its pain. Roger, for one, came to believe this was the case.

We chose to believe it, too.

BEFORE YOU GO

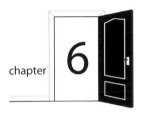

chapter 6

Eric

BEFORE YOU GO

'Say What You Need to Say'

John Mayer, in *Bucket List*

Most of us, when we come to die, won't be worried about whether we achieved enough, what we looked like, or how much stuff we acquired. We're far more likely to cling to the people we hold in our hearts, and who hold us in theirs. Just as real estate is about location, location, location, death and dying are about relationships, relationships, relationships. Hospice tells us in countless testimonies that it's people, not things, we want at the end.

But there are a few exceptions.

One case that stands out in my experience is that of Eric Kandel, a 53-year-old structural engineer and consultant felled by prostate cancer at the height of his career. From the moment of his terminal diagnosis, Eric remained in total denial of his condition. Instead, he expended much precious energy attempting to defeat every unstoppable loss, even as he seemed to lose sight altogether of his caring life partner.

Eric and his wife, Claire, who was herself a top-level corporate executive, had been married for nineteen years, without children. Both were accustomed to success and all its trappings. They lived in a high-end, high-rise condo complex—a tall, sleek building wrapped in a shiny aluminum exterior that commanded the attention of passersby. Its eleven stories of metal and glass towered over the soft brown tones and gentle sloping roofs of the brick buildings below.

I stood admiring this triumphant tower—*what a view it must command from on high!*—as Sandi, our social worker on the case, and I plugged the parking meter in the street. We were about to pay the Kandels our first joint home visit, and Sandi was prepping me about what to expect. She'd already made two solo visits to the Kandel home and had found Eric to be both moody and uncommunicative. It seemed our patient was singularly resistant to connecting with anyone attending to him.

"Don't be too surprised if he changes his mind at the last minute and doesn't want to see us, Cherí."

We paused, standing in the snow at the main entrance, while Sandi checked her notes for the combination to the security-locked door. Finding it, she punched in the numbers on the touchpad. A moment later, we were buzzed in to our patient's world.

We crossed the lobby and took the soundless elevator to the ninth floor. Our single knock on the Kandel's front door was answered by Eric's housekeeper, Marina, who warmly invited us to "come in, please." Just as we stepped inside, however, we heard Eric bark instructions to hold us there: "They'll have to wait. I want to be dressed properly."

Marina's smile vanished. She motioned for us to wait where we stood. Despite Eric's weak and nauseous condition, he would not allow himself to meet with us lying abed in his pajamas. Perhaps he'd change his mind about seeing us today after all.

After waiting a few moments in the foyer, we gained admittance to Eric's private domain. Marina led us through the spare kitchen into the spotless interior of an open living room with an efficient furniture arrangement: couch, coffee table, two chrome-trimmed leather chairs, and the upholstered chair in which Eric Kandel sat waiting—all were positioned perfectly around the perimeter of a rectangular area rug. Metal bookshelves at the end of the room held volumes of *Architectural Digest* in perfectly aligned periodical containers, each labeled by date.

Eric sat upright in a rust-brown chair, resting his feet on the matching ottoman. His appearance bespoke fastidious care and immaculate grooming—well-cut, slate-gray hair contrasting with a soft gray T-shirt, pressed jeans, white cotton socks, and cashmere slippers. His ebony-framed designer glasses broke the long lines of a still-handsome, but emaciated face.

There was no welcome. Eric scrutinized us and pointed us in the direction of the leather chairs across from him. "You can sit there," he said, breaking the silence with a slight air of annoyance. "My wife should be here soon."

For a moment I hesitated to introduce myself. Then I stepped toward him and extended my hand. "I'm Cherí Milton, Mr. Kandel, part of your care team."

Eric nodded slightly but didn't take my hand.

I nodded politely in turn. "Sandi asked me to come along today to get acquainted with you and Claire," I said. "I'll be available to offer support." My instincts told me, correctly, that Eric Kandel was not keen on the idea of talking to a *counselor*. He clearly had nothing else he wanted to say.

I took my assigned seat, glad that I'd been prepared for a cool reception, and hung back while Sandi gently queried Eric about how he was feeling. Over the months, both Sandi and Candace, the hospice nurse, had observed Eric struggle painfully with each new phase of his treatment—especially having to rely on a catheter.

Not once during that time had he expressed any feelings about his deteriorating condition, as if he believed that by refusing to recognize his symptoms, he could somehow make them go away.

Only much later did I see how the condo tower offered a perfect metaphor for Eric's resistance. Strong, unyielding, protected from outside influences, it weathered the forces of nature, day in and day out, with metallic indifference. Or so it seemed.

From where I sat with Sandi and Eric, I could easily glimpse the interior of the master bedroom. Two spacious rooms were separated by French doors swung wide open for easy movement from room to room. The bed had been made with stark white sheets, tucked in at the corners military-style. A charcoal blanket folded in thirds lay across the bottom. Pillows were stacked two high, with each edge lined up square. Identical stainless steel tables flanked the bed, with matching boxes of white tissues exactly centered on each one.

As I pondered the scene, Eric answered Sandi's questions in a low monotone. He spoke with exaggerated precision, elongating and enunciating every syllable. After each pronouncement, Sandi would attempt to repeat the essence of what she'd understood him to say. Each time he would pounce, "correcting" whatever she said with an air of contempt. His aggressive editing was embarrassing to everyone—an effect he apparently intended.

Sandy persisted in a calm tone. "So you would like the nurse to suggest something to help with your nausea?"

"*No*! I am *not* going to take any more drugs—I'm *done* with chemo!" Eric snapped. "I don't want to be nauseous; I want my body to settle down so I can eat."

"You don't want to take any more drugs," Sandi affirmed.

"I'm *not* taking any more drugs—is what I said. I should be feeling more of an appetite now. I need to eat to keep up my strength."

"I'm noting your concerns," said Sandi, jotting them down in her notebook.

"I'm not concerned," Eric retorted, rolling his eyes. "I just want to eat without throwing it all back up."

"Okay, I think I understand. I'll let Candace, your nurse, know about your nausea," Sandi offered.

"I would certainly expect you to tell her, but I also want you to tell her: *No more drugs!*"

And so went this one-sided tug-of-war. To myself I wondered about Eric having crossed the line between a fierce and justifiable need for privacy and a tyrannical obsession. He clearly perceived us as a threat, a nuisance, a waste of his time. Was there perhaps some secret code—known only to his wife or a select few—that allowed access to his locked-down world?

Despite Eric's willful efforts to recover on his terms, his cancer wasn't cooperating. In response, he doubled down on his efforts. The degree of his fixation was remarkable.

Meanwhile, Claire Kandel arrived home and joined us. She smiled "hello" and briefly laid her hands on Eric's shoulders. "I'm back, honey," she said, and then moved to take a seat next to her husband. In so doing, she bumped the coffee table, nudging it slightly forward.

Instantly, Eric readjusted it. "You shouldn't sit so close, Claire, it makes me feel claustrophobic," he said, leaning away from her.

Claire said nothing but dutifully scooted her body to the opposite end of the couch. She listened intently as Sandi and Eric concluded their exchange, neither commenting nor asking questions.

There *he* was, obsessed with the details of a treatment regimen that soon would vanish. And here *she* was, a loving, available partner. Why, we wondered, did Eric not lean on the bond with his wife—the very thing that *could* sustain him? It was frustrating.

Yet Claire was something of a mystery, too. As a corporate vice president, she knew very well how to assert herself. But she had offered no resistance when Eric pushed her to continue working. Maybe the effort of trying to manage her career and a sick husband left her exhausted. Whatever her reasons, Claire's working full-time meant Eric was largely alone.

We were surprised when, our visit concluded, Claire pursued us to the front door. "Can I speak with you a moment?" she whispered urgently.

"Of course, Claire. What's on your mind?"

She commenced to pour her heart out. "I'm having such a hard time with Eric. He controls *everything*." Tears welled in her eyes. "He just sends me off to work and won't even talk about the fact that he's dying."

"That must be painful for you."

Claire wiped her tears away. "I don't understand how he does it. He feels just *terrible*—he's *dying!* How can he think about stuff that just doesn't matter?"

"He's having an awfully hard time, isn't he?" I said.

"It's just so sad. But, you know, I can't go on like this." Her voice was full of sudden resolve. "I need to take some steps to deal with the situation, whether Eric does or not."

Right then and there, we agreed to meet at the next available opportunity to explore ways in which Claire might connect with Eric. Clearly she longed for authentic, heart-to-heart intimacy with him.

But it wasn't to be. Before we had the chance to sit down together, Eric's decline accelerated to the point he was unable to speak. Ironically, not two weeks earlier, he had canceled a follow-up visit with me, explaining that the throw rugs were in the wash and not yet ready to be put down. I might track in snow and slush from outside!

Now he was all but incapacitated.

Claire told me over the phone how she was coping. "I've

been journaling and writing letters to Eric. They say how I feel about him and what our life together has meant to me."

"That sounds like a positive step, Claire."

"But it's not enough. I need to say these things out loud, and I want someone to hear them. Do you think I could read the letters to you—is that dumb?"

"Not at all. I'd be honored. But I think you need to read them to Eric first. Even if he can't speak, most patients in his condition keep their hearing right to the end. You can still read your letters to him."

"You think so?"

"Yes, I do. Read them to Eric as soon as you can. And if you still want me to hear them after that, I'm available."

༄ ༄ ༄

It turned out that I was able to visit Eric and Claire Kandel one last time. There in the master bedroom, Eric lay on his bed like a deflated balloon, just skin and bones. He was barely responsive. Claire sat by his side, keeping vigil.

She had read all her letters to him, she told me, hoping he had understood. Yet she couldn't help but grieve the lost time with him, lost opportunities for extraordinary moments together, lost words that would never be spoken or heard. Later that day, Claire climbed in bed beside Eric, speaking aloud her thoughts to him while he faded in and out of sleep.

He died at home six days later.

A week after his death, I got a call from Claire. She sounded a bit breathless. "Cherí, I had to tell you about what happened two days after Eric died. I was on my computer looking through my old emails for a poem to use at his memorial service, and I stumbled on an old message from him—something he'd written two years ago.

She rushed ahead. "It wasn't a special occasion or anything, but for some reason he wrote me the most beautiful three-page letter. He told me how much he loved me and what I meant to him, and how I'd made his life so much better. Of course, I saved it but then somehow totally forgot about it, I don't know how. Then, last week, there it was! Can you believe the timing?"

"That's pretty amazing," I said.

"Yes! I was just stunned. I'm telling you, Cherí, when I first reread his letter and pored over the words, I could *feel* him here with me, you know? And it was all the things I wanted us to say to each other before he died."

"How sweet for you."

"It is. I believe with all my heart Eric somehow caused me to find that email. It was his message to me from heaven. It just about makes up for all those times he wouldn't talk to me."

In the end Eric's letter seemed the answer to Claire's prayers. Still and all, from my personal perspective, it seems a shame to leave a void when a powerful face-to-face moment might have happened between the Kandels.

If I've learned anything from working with people all these years, it's that each of us needs someone to witness our lives, our loves, our dreams. Even our pain needs to be heard by *someone*. As the song says, "Say what you need to say."

Allow me to share my own ideal deathbed scenario. When I lay dying, I want to gather my family and friends around me, let them climb up on the bed and surround me with their smiles, their sighs, their tears. I want them to talk to me—talk to each other—until everyone has said what they needed to say, and until I, too, have said my piece. Then we all wait together in the deepest silence of all.

BEFORE YOU GO

BEFORE YOU GO

Ricky

Ghosts Shadowing Ghosts

Each substance of a grief hath twenty shadows.

Shakespeare, in *Richard II*

When someone dies, we miss not only the person we loved but a host of intangibles—the sense of safety, security, and companionship our loved one may have represented. We experience upset in the smallest niches in our lives wherein our loved one played a role. And we miss our own roles and duties in relation to them.

Such unforeseen losses often come as a surprise.

One such loss commonly impacts long-term caregivers. When suddenly the intense burdens of caregiving are lifted from us, we expect relief. What we're unprepared to lose is the sense of structure and meaning the role of caregiver conferred on us. We even miss the intensity of the role itself.

This phenomenon is known as grieving "secondary losses," those losses a death brings in its wake. The difficult thing about such losses is that you cannot predict how they'll make themselves known. Everyday rhythms, familiar meanings, and responses shift in subtle ways, and we're suddenly aware of new "absences"—and new griefs.

That's what happened to Ricky, a quiet first grader whose 11-year-old brother Rodney lay dying in our inpatient unit after an accident.

Rodney had been transferred from the hospital setting to our facility after staff determined he was brain dead. At the family's request, life support was removed to allow for a peaceful, natural death. Nursing staff expected Rodney would die within a few hours and wished to offer the family extra support. Ricky's mom, Annette, had already given permission for me to talk with Ricky and see how he was doing.

It was late in the afternoon when I stepped into Rodney's room to find Annette and Ricky keeping a bedside vigil. Ricky sat absorbed in paging through a coloring book, his small frame swallowed up by a large recliner chair. The sight struck me as painfully funny—I couldn't help but think of *Goldilocks and the Three Bears* when she would say, "This one's too big."

Given the intensity of the situation, Ricky's preoccupation was not surprising. Annette, though, was expecting me. Dressed in blue jeans and a hooded sweatshirt, she immediately stood up from her chair and extended her hand.

"I'm so glad you're here. We've been waiting for you. Ricky, say hello to Cherí! This is the lady who's going to show you some fun stuff down the hall." Annette's shell-shocked face belied her bravado. No doubt she desperately desired a few final moments alone with her dying son.

Taking my cue, I knelt down by Ricky's chair and smiled. "Hello, Ricky! I've heard a lot about you. I guess the nurses told you about me, too?"

Ricky nodded shyly. His "hello" was barely a whisper.

"Good! They told you about our special project room for kids, right?" Time and again I'd seen how doing a small craft project with kids can work magic. Often, they open up and express their worries.

Ricky sat up straight in his chair, his brown eyes open

wide with interest. For a moment he looked over at Rodney lying motionless on the bed, and then at his mom. Annette smiled her permission. "Go ahead, honey."

"It's just down the hall, and you only have to stay as long as you want to," I reassured him.

"Okay," Ricky said. He jumped up and followed me down the hall to the children's activity room. His face brightened immediately at the sight of long shelves full of Hobby Lobby spoils. Surveying the loot, he spotted a large roll of paper and pounced on it.

"Can I use some of this to make a picture?"

"Sure! That paper's so big, you can draw whatever you want on it. What do you want to use—crayons, markers, or—" here I paused and raised my eyebrows dramatically—"*paint?*"

"Paint! I want to paint on that big paper!"

We rolled out the huge sheet and laid it on top of the newsprint covering the tabletop. Ricky helped me position the jars of poster paints at the corners where he could reach them easily.

"Can I paint whatever I want?"

"Yes, whatever you want."

"Even a word?"

"A word?" I repeated, not sure what he meant.

"Uh-huh—a word. I just want to paint a word."

"Oh, like a special message?" I wondered what inspiration had seized him.

"Umm … yeah." Ricky dipped his brush into the green paint without further explanation. He paused a moment, then very carefully made a wide green brushstroke down the paper. Soon after came a second, parallel stroke. Next he bridged the two with a horizontal swipe. He pulled back to survey the results: a giant *H*.

He emitted a small sigh of satisfaction. Dipping again into the green paint, he painstakingly sketched a giant capital

E. His lips moved as he sounded out the letters of the word he was trying to spell. "*H-E-, H-E-, H-E-, H-E-L-L,*" he whispered, and then got quiet.

Uh-oh. Where's this going? "Are you painting a message for your brother?"

Ricky ignored my question. Instead he paused, holding the brush in mid-air. His eyes moved back and forth from paint to paper. Without looking up he asked, "How do you spell *help*?"

"*Help?*" I wasn't sure I'd heard him correctly.

"Yeah—*help*—how do you spell *help*?" he repeated, staring down at the paper.

"Okay. The next letter is *L*, and then *P*." Thankfully, he wasn't spelling *hell* after all!

"Rodney always spells stuff for me," Ricky confided, giving me a glimpse of one of the special niches his brother occupied for him. Keeping his eyes on the page, and holding the brush tightly in his small hand, he painted first the letter *L*, then *P*, to complete the word *HELP*.

There it was: a single giant word with just a few scattered drops of green paint to adorn it. *HELP* took up the entire page. Ricky's green shout-out conjured the familiar predicament of a shipwreck survivor marooned on an island.

"Do you want me to get another piece of paper for you?" I thought we might need more to fill out the message.

"Nope."

"You don't want to add any more words to what you painted?"

"No, just *HELP*. That's all." Then he added a surprising request: "Can I tape it up in my brother's room right now?"

"Well, sure." I tried my best to fathom his intent. "Ricky, do you wish you could help Rodney right now?"

Ricky sighed. "No. I can't help him. You know he's gonna die, right?"

I was humbled. It dawned on me that for once it was *Ricky's* turn to tell someone the overwhelming news, "Rodney is dying."

"Yes, I know," I said solemnly. "Can I ask you something, Ricky?"

"Yeah. Okay."

"Was Rodney someone who would help *you*?"

Ricky nodded and dunked his paintbrush into the water cup for cleaning. He was done talking and painting. "Can we go hang this up now?"

"Almost—it's got a little more drying to do. Let's try this," I said, fanning the sign to speed-dry it. Ricky could barely wait. Soon he swiped his finger across the sign and pronounced it "dry enough."

With sign and masking tape in hand, we headed straight back to Rodney's room and posted *HELP* over his bed. Annette watched it all without saying a word.

Rodney died not longer after. He slipped away with his mom and Ricky lying in bed next to him. A few close relatives had also gathered to say their goodbyes.

☙ ☙ ☙

Two weeks after Rodney's funeral, the social worker asked if I could please check in with Ricky at home. Annette was worried that he'd become very quiet. Was he doing okay? She really wanted our opinion before sending him back to first grade.

I knocked on the door of Annette and Ricky's apartment instead of pressing the badly cracked doorbell patched with tape. Annette's haggard face at the door wasn't as shocking as the change evident in her whole bearing. Although probably in her late thirties, she looked much older—like an aging rag doll, shoulders slumped, arms hanging in place without energy or movement.

She showed me into the living room, where Ricky sat on the floor surrounded by new toys from extended family. He was bright eyed and well rested—just the opposite of his mom.

Annette excused herself in a flat voice. "I'm going to the kitchen to put away the groceries and do the dishes."

Ricky scrutinized me for a moment. "I remember you. You let me paint a picture for Rodney's room."

"That's right, Ricky," I settled myself on the floor next to him. "We hung up your green *HELP* sign in Rodney's room."

"Yeah, but I don't know what happened to it. I think my mom's got it with some other stuff."

I nodded, and went straight to the heart of the matter. "Ricky, I'm so sorry that Rodney died."

He nodded nonchalantly. Not much of an opening.

"How was Rodney's funeral?" I asked.

"It lasted too long. It was kinda boring," he said hesitantly, not sure if he was allowed to call a funeral boring. Many children have pronounced the same opinion to me over the years, and I always appreciated their frankness.

As Ricky added nothing else, I tried turning the conversation in another direction. "I was wondering, what's changed around here since Rodney died—anything?"

"Uhm, noffing."

"I bet you miss your big brother."

"Um, I dunno." He let out a grunt of frustration, picking up a loose part belonging to one of his newly assembled race cars. He seemed far more interested in playing than in answering my questions.

I decided to ask one more question that's often helpful in these situations. "Ricky, is there anything you're afraid of since Rodney died?"

Without hesitation, he answered, "Yes!" as if I had just poked the very secret he wanted to share.

"I'm not surprised," I said. "Lots of kids tell me that."

He didn't look up.

"What is it you're afraid of since Rodney died?" I asked softly, fully expecting him to tell me he was afraid someone else close to him might die—a common worry for a child his age.

"I'm afraid I'll be late for school, and then I'll be in trouble."

Oh! I was bemused. How did this fear relate to Rodney's death? Ricky's downcast expression showed just how much he worried about getting into trouble at school.

"You're afraid you'll be late for school? Why do you think so?"

"Um," said Ricky, struggling to put the right words together. "Every day we get ready for school, and Rodney and me go outside to get on our bus, right down there by that blue house." He jumped up and pointed out the window.

I got up, too, and looked out with him. The blue house was visible halfway down the block. "I see it."

Suddenly the tears came. "There's like, lots of buses that stop, and they're 'zackly alike. Rodney always tells me which one is the right bus for me to get on. Now I'm gonna get on the *wrong* bus."

All of this little boy's worry and sadness came tumbling out. "My teacher will yell at me for coming in late." His chin quivered. "I'll be in trouble." Ricky had lost not only his big brother but his morning bus coach.

What other terrors might be haunting him?

My heart broke to see how he struggled all alone with his dilemma. I wanted to scoop him up and assure him that no one could possibly yell at him for being late to school. *One hopes!* At least I could reassure him that someone would gladly help him find the right bus in the morning. It was a start.

Once again, I was struck by how powerful are the unforeseen ways in which we—especially children—can experience a loved one's absence. Since encountering Ricky's story of "sideways grief," his poignant *HELP* message has resonated deeply in my heart. What a perfect symbol for grief's ripple effects!

Ricky's message calls on us to respect the unforeseen shadows that grief can cast over our lives. It reminds us we can offer each other a most gracious gift by patiently acknowledging the need every one of us has to grieve in our own way, on our own timetable.

BEFORE YOU GO

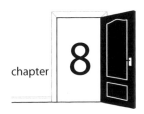

chapter 8

Marvin

Just Be There

A loving silence often has far more power to heal and to connect than the most well-intentioned words.

Rachel Remen

It's a challenge when someone we care about is experiencing difficulty and we want to "help fix it." But there is no fix. We feel compelled to act, to call someone or do something—anything—to bring resolution. Yet there's nothing we can do.

My work with hospice patients and families has taught me that we still can offer something very powerful to these situations. Being wholly present with someone in crisis, willing to listen to their thoughts and feelings—without voicing expectations or judgments, pronouncing solutions, or taking any action whatsoever—can have a real, healing impact.

Silent listening may be the most powerful action we can take. We simply offer our attitude of kindness and compassion toward another human being.

All that's required is our coming to the situation with hearts open and guards down. Regardless of another's ability to communicate, we can bring comfort and nurture their soul by just being there in their hour of need.

Marvin Holden was 89 years old. He had resided in an assisted living complex for many years, in his own tiny apartment. A long-time machinist in a local factory, Marvin was forced to retire when doctors diagnosed him with cardiac myopathy, or severe heart failure. Still, he was intent on staying busy and worked part-time in the mailroom of a local nonprofit agency. He sorted the mail, made deliveries, and socialized with the maintenance crew. But the day came when his deteriorating heart condition compelled him to quit.

Though unsteady on his feet, and under the watchful eye of staff, Marvin walked proudly without assistance. He would lumber down the hall, dragging along his six-foot-three-inch frame and joshing with every nursing assistant along the way. He loved to connect with the staff, finding new ways to tease them every day. Naturally, his smiling, good humor endeared him.

Marvin would start each day by making his own breakfast. Then he would climb the steps to the "memory care ward" on the second floor where his wife, Arlene, occupied a room. For many years, she had suffered with Alzheimer's disease and now required constant care. Though she did not recognize Marvin, he spent much of each day keeping her company and assisting with her meals.

Unlike Arlene, Marvin was blessed with a mind that stayed sharp right up to the final days of his life. Besides teasing everybody, his other passion was his faith. He attended Sunday services whenever he could get a ride to church, and his conversation was peppered with references to the Good Book and the Golden Rule.

One Saturday, Marvin didn't show up for lunch in the dining hall. Staff hastened to his room to look for him. They found him still lying in bed sleeping. To their dismay, he declined each attempt to wake him, even to eat. As he grew less and less responsive, they worried about losing him.

For two days he ate nothing, spoke hardly a word, and slept around the clock. Staff felt compelled to notify Arlene and Marvin's only son, Peter, of Marvin's unresponsive condition. Although Peter lived with his family within manageable driving distance, he had seldom, if ever, visited. When contacted about his dad's rapid decline, he was surprisingly unmoved.

Even when staff voiced their concerns more urgently—Marvin might be near death, they cautioned—Peter remained unflappable: "My current job commitments won't allow me to get away for two days at least."

Was it just willful denial? Did he not care? Again, staff urged an immediate family visit. Again, Peter insisted that neither he nor his wife, Flora, could get away for at least two more days. He did, however, request that his dad be admitted to hospice. "Also," he pressed, "could you please notify my mother that Marvin is sick?"

Staff grumbled their disappointment. It looked like Marvin, whom they cared about deeply, would die alone. His few living friends were physically unable to visit him, and now his family was deserting him!

In the end, staff had to allow family dynamics to be what they were. Maybe Peter was overwhelmed by denial—or by guilt. Or maybe—though this seemed unlikely—there was some shadowy history of abuse behind the family estrangement. No one knew.

Staff proceeded to comply with Peter's request to admit his father to hospice—conferring with Marvin's primary physician, arranging the paperwork, and formally obtaining Peter's verbal consent. Their final act of care for Marvin was to arrange for his transport to our inpatient unit.

He arrived Monday evening, unaccompanied by anyone near or dear. The nurses could only make sure he was as comfortable as possible and attempt to find a volunteer to spend an hour or two at his bedside.

As it happened, no one was able to help out on such short notice, and Marvin lay alone in his room throughout the night, still unresponsive. The only life stirring around him were the comings and goings of our staff

When I arrived at work Tuesday morning, one of the staff quickly brought Marvin's plight to my attention. My first order of the day was to check with the nurse on duty about his situation.

"How's he doing, Janice?"

"Still unresponsive. It's so sad he's in there all alone."

"It really is. Any family supposed to show up today?"

Janice hesitated. "They said this afternoon sometime. I just hope he can hang on till they get here."

"Me, too," I said, checking my calendar. "Hmm … my morning's pretty open. I could spend an hour or so with him."

Janice beamed her relief. "That'd be great! He's down in Room 26."

"Let me just grab a cup of coffee."

It was 7:30 a.m. Sunlight shone softly into Marvin's room, filtering through the white window blinds. One of the staff, noting "Pt. devoted churchgoer" in his chart, had started a CD of instrumental hymns for him. The soft music cast a soothing spell. I sat down to keep Marvin company for a while and sipped my morning coffee.

How isolated he looked! No personal effects surrounded him—no pictures, cards, or items of clothing, no empty cups left behind by visitors the day before. Even the medicine bottles had been put away. Only a handful of staff came and went, performing their routine care.

Thank goodness he was feeling no pain, I thought. He lay slightly on his left side with the bed sheet pulled up over his body, his long arms extended outside it. His translucent skin was peppered with age spots, bruises, and moles. A few strands of hair stuck to his nearly bald head, and white stubble covered his hollow cheeks.

Marvin's mouth hung slightly open. With each labored breath there was a slight pause until the next one came—a common sign of approaching death.

My relief at finding him so quiet was mixed with a measure of sadness. I would not be able to ask him how he was feeling—Was he at peace with everything? Any unfinished business to attend to?

But it wasn't about words at this point.

Twenty minutes passed as I reflected quietly and did my best to send Marvin thoughts of peace, dignity, and kindness. I mused for a moment. Was there any other way to let him know he wasn't alone? Anything else that might touch his spirit?

An inspiration seized me. I knew about Marvin's religious devotion. We were already enveloped in church music. Maybe I could sing a few old hymns for him?

I leaned over and spoke into his ear. "Good morning, Marvin. My name is Cherí, and I'm here to help take care of you. I know your faith is very, very important to you—the nurses told me. I think I can remember some old hymns from my childhood, and I'd like to try to sing them for you. Maybe you'll recognize some of them."

Marvin gave no indication he heard me.

I took hold of his hand. Clearing my throat, I began to sing. With little effort my alto voice carried the words of my first choice, "Blessed assurance, Jesus is mine, oh what a foretaste of glory divine ..." Surprisingly I remembered all the words to the first and last verses.

One by one, I introduced each new hymn I was about to sing: *Great Is Thy Faithfulness*, *Amazing Grace*, *How Great Thou Art*. Sweet melodies and honeyed words I hadn't sung in twenty years floated up from the depths of memory and flowed to Marvin.

"Do you remember these old hymns, Marvin? I think *Great is Thy Faithfulness* is my favorite. I love the phrase, 'Morning by morning new mercies I see,' don't you?" I squeezed his hand with gentle pressure. "Do you see new mercies on this beautiful sunny morning, Marvin?"

No response but a few slight twitches and a single muffled groan.

Words from another favorite hymn rose up: *I Need Thee Every Hour.* This one was composed back in 1872 by Annie Hawks. I began to sing what seemed the most fitting verse, "I need Thee every hour, oh blessed Lord I pray ..." Stroking Marvin's hand, I continued softly, "in joy or in pain come quickly and abide, or life is in vain."

Raising my voice slightly, I sang the chorus, "I need Thee, Oh I need Thee, every hour I need Thee, oh bless me now my savior I come to Thee." Keeping my eyes on Marvin, I reprised the soothing words: "I need Thee, every hour I need ..."

Marvin's brow furrowed. His lips moved, making a barely audible sound. "Thee," he whispered, finishing the phrase with me. Was it my imagination, or was he trying to sing with me?

He was! As I reprised the chorus, "Oh I need Thee, every hour I need Thee," his quiet, labored words fell into sync with my own. With Marvin following along with me, I slowed at the last phrase, "Oh bless me now my savior, I ... come ... to ... Thee."

This time it was Marvin who squeezed my hand. A single tear trickled down his cheek.

Something deep and holy was happening. Somehow I'd been privy to a private conversation between an old saint and his God. I will never forget the power of that moment.

"Thank you, Marvin," I said, choking back my tears. "Thank you for letting me sing to you, and for singing along with me."

Marvin did not speak or sing again after that. But he didn't leave us just yet. He waited until the next day and then passed peacefully—shortly after his son Peter and family had arrived and said their goodbyes.

The timing was his own.

BEFORE YOU GO

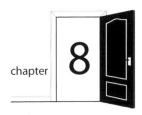

chapter 8

Lori

Growing Wings in Freefall

Understand that the right to choose
your own path is a sacred privilege.
Dwell in possibility.

Oprah Winfrey

So could Oprah be wrong? "Choose our own path ... Dwell in possibility" are surely laudable goals, ones that resonate with our human yearning to lead fulfilling lives. Naturally, we want to instill the same goals in our children. When it comes to raising them to be successful, independent adults, quite a few of us—myself included—have leaned heavily on the popular prescription: "Give them roots and wings."

Fortunately, most of us get enough of both to find our way. Our children, too. With respect to the Davis family, however, the old formula seems to have gone awry. Never have I encountered anything quite like them in my twenty-five years of counseling and hospice work!

Here was a close-knit group of singularly talented adults who, when confronted by the biggest crisis of their family life, showed themselves to be—well—let's just say, root-bound! They presented one of the most difficult puzzles our hospice team has encountered.

The family included our patient, Lori, her husband, David, a high-level executive, and the couple's three twenty-something children: Crystal, Connie, and Colin. To the outside world, all of the Davises appeared to be high-functioning, career-minded strivers. But Lori's impending death from ovarian cancer had thrown the entire family into a morass of grief, conflict, and paralysis. They were barely functioning, unable to negotiate the most basic tasks and decisions.

As soon became clear, Lori functioned as the source of all comfort, reassurance, and decisive direction for her family. She was the sun in their private solar system, and she beamed her powerful, guiding light into the far corners of their lives—providing all the answers, the right moves, the next steps each member needed to take.

At any time, should any family member tip into uncertainty or imbalance, Lori was right there to sooth, encourage, coo over, and prop up the needy one until the ground was once again firm.

This system was working well for them all until cancer arrived to eclipse their sun. Without Lori to ground them, the family's anxiety level shot off the charts. Predictably, everyone regressed quickly into serious dysfunction and raw dependence.

Now they argued about how to proceed after Lori's death. Should Dad keep the house? Who had the best claim to this or that treasured keepsake? Would Lori expect them to continue on the path she had steered them along? On and on. Each and all insisted their ideas or opinions were the right ones—the exact ones Lori would have expressed.

This was the juncture at which I was called in to help. "This family is unraveling," Sheryl, the RN case manager, told me. "Everyone's at the house now, and they're absolutely inconsolable—crying and arguing. Just really stuck! Is there any way you can come and help me out here?"

"Let me check. I think so," I said.

"Oh, that's great!" Sheryl sighed with relief. Then she added, "You know, you might want to bring another grief counselor along with you so you can tag team this family."

"Wow! The situation must be escalated," I said—which was teamspeak for "The **** must have hit the fan!" The request for two grief counselors was highly unusual. "I'll see who else is free," I promised. "Why don't you go ahead and tell the family we'll be there later this afternoon, around three or so."

"Thank you, thank you, Cherí! This is the most intense family situation I've ever dealt with. Wait'll you see—everybody's squeezed into the bedroom, crying, arguing, refusing to leave their mom's bedside!"

Admittedly, I liked the idea of tag teaming this one. Without too much trouble, I was able to secure the help of another grief counselor named Kris. We conferred and agreed she would focus her efforts on Lori and David, and I would focus mine on the "kids"—if this proved the right way to proceed.

We both knew things could go in a completely different direction in a heartbeat, and we wanted to "meet" the Davises wherever they were emotionally, spiritually, and physically.

To help us navigate "the most intense situation" the nurse had ever seen, we scooped up an armful of basic hospice literature on our way out the door—popular flyers with titles like "Anticipating Grief," "When You Lose a Parent," and "Signs of Approaching Death." Even such basic information can bring relief to survivors.

🕊 🕊 🕊

Kris and I found the impressive, two-story Davis home in an upscale neighborhood.

We knocked once lightly on the front door and let ourselves in, knowing the family would be with Lori upstairs. Just inside, we encountered Lori's husband, David, descending the stairs, looking distraught and exhausted. He came down to meet us in stained blue jeans and bare feet, his black hair uncombed.

We made our introductions. "Thank you for coming by," David said with a slight smile. "Come on upstairs. Lori's awake for now and we're just hanging out." As we followed behind him, David turned to us midstairs and said, "I warn you, we're all pretty emotional. Hope that's okay."

Kris and I reassured David that whatever he and the family were experiencing was totally okay. Because it was. I told him we'd be surprised if they weren't all "pretty emotional," emphasizing the word *surprised*. "We're used to lots of emotion, believe me."

We entered the crowded master bedroom to find family members seated on kitchen chairs surrounding Lori's bed, looking shell-shocked. The youngest two children, Crystal, 23, and Colin, 25, hovered together in the farthest corner of the room talking in hushed voices, while the oldest daughter, Connie, sat across the room talking softly with her grandmother, Lori's mom. Lori's dad and sister were there, too. They sat totally erect, not saying a word.

Lori lay in the middle of a floral-print bedspread, dressed in sweat pants, a zip-up hoodie, and slippers. Her short, sandy-blonde hair, cut pixie style, accentuated her pretty face and hollow cheeks. She lay very still, her eyes open.

David climbed up beside her and began gently stroking her hair. With his free hand, he patted the corner of the bed and said to Kris and me, "You two can sit here. It's okay. Really."

We did as David directed, although a little reluctantly. Always we wanted to respect the personal space of our patients. In any case, Lori didn't seem to mind, and she managed to give us a genuine smile.

The family fell silent as we sat down.

"We know this is a terribly difficult situation for all of you," I began. "It's evident how much you love Lori. I'm sure you never expected in a million years to have to think about her dying so young."

Lori's mom nodded grimly. I looked from one to another of the Davises. "Tell us about how today has gone for you all," I continued. "I understand from your nurse, Sheryl, that things have been pretty intense, and …"

Crystal, the youngest, cut me off: "You have no idea—this is just a mess. They're saying mom maybe has two more months to live. But she promised to help me get my first teaching job. She can't just die now. We need her—I need her."

Colin, who looked like a younger version of his dad, spoke up. "I live on the East Coast, but I check in with my mom every day. She's the one I call when I miss home." His voice broke. "How can I live so far away if she's not even here?"

The others remained silent, and David seemed to be staring off in the opposite direction. "What are you thinking, David?" I said, trying to pull him back. "Do you have a response to Crystal and Colin's comments?"

David turned to face me. "Lori's the glue of this family," he said, fighting back tears. "She holds all of us together—including me. How can we get along without her?" He closed his eyes. "Why couldn't it be me instead?"

"I'm sorry, honey," Lori murmured. The anguish in the room was palpable.

Connie finally broke the silence. "Ah, mom, who's going to plan our vacations now?" she asked half teasing, half lamenting. "You always made it all work somehow. We don't even know where to start." She hastened to explain to Kris and me that the whole family—some twenty people—were accustomed to taking vacations together. "We've gone to a tropical island every year since I was born."

She shook her head at David. "This whole thing is just unbelievable, Dad."

I listened, a little shocked, as one after another of the Davises voiced their incredulity and refusal to accept the situation. Yet was I mistaken, or had Lori all but apologized for dying just now? Was anyone in this family capable of putting her needs first at this critical time?

It was unsettling. Maybe, I thought, the very fact that Lori had been in and out of remission for several years—she was still working outside the home only weeks before—led them to assume she would rebound once again.

In any case, as a former family counselor, I saw that the Davises (probably early on) must have locked into a pretty elementary level of functioning. It was all about staying dependent on mom. Lori's executive radiance overshadowed each family member's growth into autonomy. Her children had been born into it, and her husband had come to depend on it completely.

As I was to learn in follow-up sessions with him, David was inclined to be quick tempered, and relied on Lori to "manage him." Now he was overwhelmed, a deer in the headlights.

In fact, Lori had functioned as arbiter for the whole family, whose style of communication was really arguing. All the Davises were strong, opinionated personalities who held each other to impossibly high standards. As a result, they blew up at each other continually. At one point, Connie observed, "We're a crazy family when we should be supporting each other."

Right! I was quickly drafted to fill the role of chief soother and final arbiter. "As terrible as this situation is, other families have experienced it, too," I assured the Davises. "You'll get through it."

Meanwhile, I encouraged them to focus on making Lori's final days good ones. After all, she was the one dying. We could sort out the other stuff later.

Lori's death came within a month, sooner than anyone envisioned. During much of that time, she was unresponsive and unaware of the waves of panic that rippled through her family.

She died peacefully at home one sunny morning, with David lying beside her and the children surrounding her bedside.

Following Lori's death, the family continued to need plenty of support. I saw the Davises many times on a one-to-one basis (or consulted with them by phone). They also participated in separate grief groups, which hospice recommends for up to a year after losing a loved one.

Although the family continued to struggle through much conflict and confusion, they also grew emotionally. Colin, Crystal, and Connie Davis found their own strength and competence learning to care for Lori. They began to trust they could apply the same skills to their own lives and loves.

My job as they tested their new wings was to listen, listen, listen. To encourage them to fully express their grief and loss, but also to identify their own greatest challenges and strengths.

In a real way, the entire family had to fast forward through a dual challenge course: growing up and grieving all at once. It was bound to be a drawn-out process, with plenty of backsliding. To staff, even the smallest positive responses represented real progress. Over time we saw more and more glimmers of hope, more inklings of independent decision making.

Lo and behold, the Davis children began to "dwell in possibility." Crystal secured a good teaching position and managed to set up her own classroom. Connie took a big step and got married. Colin returned to the East Coast and developed his career without the regular calls to his mom.

David struggled hardest to regain his bearings. Early on, he confessed to wandering around the house and pacing for hours at a time, obsessing over how to spend his weekend or whether to contact old friends. Eventually even he began to take some decisive steps. He made the effort to reconnect with friends and—two years after Lori's death—was able to have coffee with a single woman friend without feeling guilty. He also sold the house.

While his children didn't much care for these developments, they did accept them. For the Davis family to support one another without being fused at the family hip signaled a major accomplishment, as well as an opening into possibility. While no one willingly chooses such "catastrophic growth," if you asked them today, the Davises would acknowledge their lives had expanded in unforeseen ways.

I like to think Lori was watching it all with approval.

BEFORE YOU GO

BEFORE YOU GO

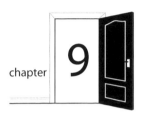

Liz

BEFORE YOU GO

We're Built for Overcoming

Although the world is full of suffering,
it is also full of the overcoming of it.

Helen Keller

Over the years, working with hospice patients and their families, I have learned just how resilient human beings can be. We don't give ourselves enough credit for this. The capacity to survive and move through the most awful, life-constricting realities is remarkable.

I've heard so many stories of individuals who, before becoming terminally ill, suffered every variety of trauma, loss, and illness, yet despite it all found a way "to fight another day." Faced with their final challenge, they sometimes broke through to a deeper experience of their own humanity and, often, renewed bonds with loved ones. But sometimes they just kept on keeping on, because that was all they knew how to do.

Liz, a young woman dying of AIDS, was one of these unblinking "survivors." During the months she was a hospice patient, she shared much of her story with me. The more I learned about the path she'd traveled, the more amazed I was by the depth of her aloneness—which was matched only by her core strength and determination. She had guts!

I first met Liz when Kristin, our RN case manager, invited me to accompany her on a check-in visit to Liz at home only three weeks after she entered outpatient hospice. At this point I had not yet been involved in direct care for any of our AIDS patients. Kristin and I did know, however, that Liz expressed no interest in pastoral counseling or grief support during the intake process. Nor did she want any outreach to family or friends.

Because Liz was so young—only 32—and dying of AIDS during a time when the disease was mostly treatable (the mid-2000s), I was curious about her history, about which the caseworker's notes said little. (This is due partly to hospice's concern for patient privacy.)

How had she fallen through the cracks? Why had her AIDS not been treated with new, life-sustaining interventions?

I was to learn that, sadly, Liz had not sought help for her AIDS early enough to arrest it and prevent a succession of secondary infections. She was not alone in making this fatal mistake: As of this writing, it's estimated over 200,000 Americans diagnosed with AIDS have chosen not to enter treatment. They may feel too well, or find the medical system too daunting, or fear the stigma. We don't know all the reasons.

So Liz and her AIDS had fought each other without quarter. By the time I encountered her, the disease had taken its final, devastating turn. Now, given her death sentence, we were left wondering why, oh why, was this young woman choosing to die without a single friend or family member nearby?

Kristin and I climbed to the second floor of a subsidized apartment complex, one of many in a low-income neighborhood. We knocked at Liz's door and waited, knowing she needed time to get to the door. After a few minutes, we heard the lock disengage, but she didn't open the door for us. Instead she returned immediately to her landing pad, the sofa, and sank down again.

"Come in—the door's open," she called to us.

At this point, I knew little about what to expect. So I was pretty shocked when we stepped inside Liz's apartment. Here were stacks and stacks of papers, magazines, and catalogs in ragged columns, some touching the ceiling, as well as endless piles of small boxes, assorted packages, and discarded items.

It was wall-to-wall chaos.

Later we would learn Liz had purchased many, many items from the home shopping network. Sometimes she would open a package when it arrived but not remove the contents. Other times, she removed the contents but abandoned new items on the spot. They lay where she dropped them.

Liz's small apartment also featured three bulging, black bags of garbage and heaping mounds of laundry crammed into the corners. The top of her kitchen table was just visible above the sea of refuse. It, too, was piled high with dusty books and dirty dishes.

As we made our way across the kitchen, we had to navigate around several small bowls bearing remnants of cat food, and two more filled with water. From the corner of my eye I saw the sink area was overflowing with more dirty dishes. A tiny pile of cat feces adorned a corner of the countertop. Yikes! Did I even want to know what might lie behind the closed bedroom door?

Kristin and I exchanged glances.

Stepping carefully, we made our way across the living room. I was doing my best to block out the suffocating clutter and focus on Liz. She looked so tired and sick! She lay there on the sofa dressed in maroon sweat pants and an old T-shirt, her skeletal form all too visible beneath the baggy clothes. Her long, scrawny arms were crossed and resting on her stomach.

A bony right hand hung limply from her fragile wrist. Under one shirt sleeve, the bottom portion of an old tattoo was exposed—a sad reminder of vanished youth and health.

Liz's long brown hair was gathered up and fixed with a hairclip atop her head. Her gaunt face was dotted with pale freckles, and a pair of wire-rimmed glasses, their lenses smudged, sat astride her thin, hooked nose.

One physical feature literally stood out. In striking contrast with her emaciated body, Liz's breasts were implausibly huge and upright. As she lay on her back, they protruded straight up under her T-shirt like twin missiles. The sight of them brought to mind an antique tailor's dummy with wire curves. *Breast implants?* I wondered. Later, Kristin would confirm this to be case.

How ironic that these artificial body parts would endure as the only physical portion of Liz immune to disintegration by AIDS—her one visible legacy.

I hung back and tried not to stare, although Liz seemed to take no notice of my presence. She gazed up at Kristin and asked in a casual tone, "So how much do you think I weigh?"

"Well, I don't know today exactly, Liz," Kristin replied. "I didn't bring my scale this time, but last visit you weighed just about a hundred pounds." She paused. "Do you think you've lost some weight since then?"

"Yeah, I think so." Liz responded matter-of-factly.

"How have you been feeling? Any new concerns?" asked Kristin.

"Um—no. I'm tired, but I think I'll feel better when the weather turns warm again. I hate when it's cloudy!" She sighed and let go a long, weary breath.

Kristin began to check Liz's vital signs one by one, jotting notes on her pad. Liz lay quietly with her eyes closed. I still hung back, hesitant to say anything until Kristin introduced me. This she now hastened to do, quietly explaining to Liz who I was and why I was there—to listen and give support—should she want it.

Liz didn't respond.

Clearing my throat, I softly added, "Liz, you don't have to talk to me. I'm available, though, just in case. I'm here to support patients and their families. Maybe there's someone else you'd rather talk with …"

"No, I have no one, really. The only family is my cousin, Ava. She lives in Florida," Liz said, as if that was that. She said nothing more. Not wanting to press her in any way, I let the matter drop. "If it's okay, I'll leave my business card and number here for you, Liz," I said, holding up the card with a smile.

She didn't object. I laid the card on the coffee table, alongside the pill bottles, used tissues, and scraps of paper. "Don't hesitate to call me if you ever want to."

So this would be a short visit. Kristen packed her notebook and blood pressure cuff into her nursing bag, and we got up to leave. At that moment, Liz suddenly reached for a nearby bed pillow and propped herself up. She obviously wanted to say something and blinked as if to focus.

She began a rambling story in a voice betraying little emotion. "My mom left me and my sister when we were little kids. My dad raised us mostly, but he lost his job when I was in middle school. We were homeless until I went to live with my aunt. I got in trouble in high school and my aunt kicked me out, so I lived on the streets and worked … My dad never really checked in on me. Then I got AIDS. He and I had a big argument, and we don't talk anymore."

Liz paused. "I guess I don't really have any family for you to contact." Then she added with resignation, "I had a boyfriend, but he committed suicide. Since I got sick, I don't have any friends. When I couldn't go out anymore, everyone else just kinda moved on."

I listened without comment. This was a raw soul. I waited for Liz to gather herself and share more. But as suddenly as she'd begun talking, she stopped. She scooted her body down off the pillow and again lay flat on her back. Closing her eyes, she turned away and faced the back of the sofa. Clearly the visit was over.

This was to be Liz's pattern of communication. From time to time, she'd share a sudden rush of thoughts and biographical facts in her flat, reporter style, and then fall silent again.

At those times, my head would spin with the struggle to absorb so much deep, painful information. Liz would recount piece after piece of tragic personal history without emotion or insight, as if noting so many items rolling off a conveyor belt. One potent fact after another hardly seemed to register with her.

I glanced over to Kristin. How much of this did she already know? Kristin only raised her eyebrows and nodded slightly. Yes, she'd heard pieces of Liz's story before.

After a long moment, Kristin said, "Okay then, Liz. If there's nothing else, we'll say goodbye and let ourselves out."

Liz gave no indication she'd heard.

Not quite ready to leave it there, I asked, "Would it be okay if I come back sometime, Liz?"

A silent pause followed. "Sure," she whispered.

With that, Kristin and I gingerly made our way back through the chaos to the front door. Outside in the hallway, I spoke first. "She's so alone. No wonder she hoards stuff."

"Yeah, I know—it's really sad. Her bedroom's even worse—she can't even get to her bed, it's so full of junk. But as long as nobody's in any danger, we don't have to report it to anyone. The way I see it, she's dying, and there's nothing more the doctors can do for her. I can't see any good in forcing her to do something about her apartment, can you? And I don't know anyone else who would do it for her, frankly."

Reluctantly, I had to agree. Nobody was being hurt. Liz's "junk" seemed to bring her some measure of comfort and satisfaction. Surely she was entitled to that much.

"Do you think it's all true, Kristin—everything she told us about her life? It's almost too awful to believe."

"As best I can tell, it's true. She told me the same thing, and she's been pretty consistent about her facts. I think getting AIDS was the final blow in her relationships. She told me when her dad found out about it, he never spoke to her again. A few weeks ago her cousin Ava told him Liz was dying, and he still hasn't made any contact." Apparently, Ava herself had no plans to make the trip from Florida to Wisconsin.

My heart could only go out to Liz. When I would arrive, she'd be lying on the sofa, not saying a word, when suddenly some new, horrific detail about her life would come tumbling out: She'd been abused physically by the man married to her aunt. She'd been raped when she lived on the streets. She'd gone hungry many times and waited beside a restaurant dumpster to get discarded food.

There was never a pause to reflect. Liz didn't seem to hold a grudge against anyone, and she never bemoaned her ill fortune. Oddly, the most emotion she ever expressed was anger toward the restaurant that went out of business and took away her easy access to food.

At one point, I was moved to ask how she had managed to survive such a harrowing set of life circumstances. "I don't know how I survived," she shrugged. "I've never really thought about it. I guess I didn't have a choice. I just did what I had to do to get through it." No inspirational motivation; it was a simple matter of self-preservation. Her unbending stance reminded me of Mary, the elderly patient who insisted on dying sitting up. (Mary's story starts on page 21.)

Like Mary, Liz seemed to fit the textbook model of "survivor," one simply driven to prevail, like an Energizer® bunny defying a hostile world. One who never learned to trust or rely on others. Tragically, as with Mary, Liz's grit in the face of adversity seemed to come at the cost of living without joy, love, or comfort.

This was a life painful to imagine! If only Liz could have lived long enough to use her wonderful, desperate strength to heal her life. She might have found some stability, and possibly one day created a family of own. Instead, she was destined to miss out on even the most basic experiences of her own generation. This would be her end: to die completely alone, ravaged by disease. It didn't seem fair.

However much Liz might have cooperated with her fate, the stigma of AIDS seemed to keep her family and friends at a distance. As a result, she both sought and experienced ever-increasing isolation.

Toward the end, even those of us on her care team had to keep our distance. Because Liz developed an open wound, we were obliged to take extreme precautions around her. During my last two visits, I had to wear a mask and gloves. This measure actually offered one positive—for me. The mask served to hide my deep personal sadness from Liz, and this let me be a bit braver about asking the hard questions when the moment came.

"Liz, do you think about dying? How do you feel about what's going on?"

"I know am going to die soon, and it's okay. I'm okay with it," Liz responded wearily. She would get through her dying the same way she'd gotten through everything else life had thrown at her! No fuss, no panic, no recriminations. It was what it was; just get through it.

Surely there's a better way! Buddhist teacher Pema Chodron has written, "Only to the extent that we expose ourselves over and over to annihilation can that which is indestructible in us be found." But only if we're looking for it, we might be tempted to add. All the great spiritual traditions teach us that it's through crisis and heartbreak that the soul grows and finds the path to healing.

Liz had her share of both, and yet it seemed not much light had penetrated her life. She had plenty of guts but allowed herself little glory. Is that not a double tragedy?

BEFORE YOU GO

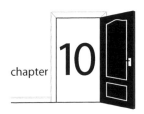

Bob

Peace, Only Peace

Be at peace with your own soul, then heaven and earth will be at peace with you.

St. Jerome

While doing hospice work I have admired those patients who find great peace and are unafraid to die. Some find a sense of serenity in appreciation for the long life they've enjoyed. Some acquire it through the love and support of their family or through pastoral counseling.

Some anticipate such blessed relief from their pain and suffering that they welcome the end with resolve and acceptance.

But there are a few patients who truly and gratefully anticipate "what's to come." They look forward to it with a sense of wonder and awe, as confident of the outcome as a starving man about to taste his first bite at the banquet table.

Bob Christiansen was such a man. I met 74-year-old Bob, a retired carpenter and cabinet maker, and his wife, Laura, on our inpatient unit. Bob had managed his pancreatic cancer well for three years with excellent medical intervention, but now the disease was rapidly metastasizing throughout his body.

Once doctors assured him there was nothing else they could do for him, Bob opted for hospice care sooner rather than later. Having recently had a close friend die in hospice, he was familiar with our services. He also very much wanted Laura to have all the support she needed.

For us, Bob's having signed on to hospice early in his end-of-life process represented the ideal. Not only did his timely admission allow the care team ample opportunity to get to know him and Laura, it meant he would still be strong enough to get around. As he remained in his home early on, he could visit with friends and family at will, as well as communicate his thoughts and wishes clearly.

Bob's team was able to learn about the things that mattered most to him and his family. They knew his greatest wish was to remain at home and die, with his wife and daughter at his side.

At the time I met the Christiansens, Bob's in-home nurse had recommended he be admitted to the inpatient unit (IPU) for a full assessment of the intense pain he was experiencing. This way, the hospice doctors and pharmacist could identify and prescribe an appropriate medication cocktail to bring him maximum relief.

The goal was clear: Get Bob's pain under control so he could return home as soon as possible.

It was on Bob's third day in the IPU that I stopped by to meet him and Laura. As I approached his room, I was surprised to hear cheerful voices. Although we often have families and patients express some measure of contentment, and even joy, they rarely do so in voices as animated as these!

Entering the room I was met by a wave of calm. What did Bob and Laura Christiansen know that I didn't?

Laura squeezed my hand in greeting. "Well, it's just so nice to meet you, Cherí! Everyone's been just wonderful, and Bob's feeling so much better!" The youthful twinkle in Laura's bright-blue eyes belied the white hair and matronly bearing. But her face was drawn, testifying to the past two nights spent on the fold-out couch in Bob's room. She didn't want to miss a single minute of the time she had left with him.

In fact, Bob looked much more rested than his wife. Thank goodness the new medication was working. Now Laura needed to get some rest.

"It makes such a difference to feel comfortable, doesn't it?" I said, turning to Bob and extending my hand. He bore a striking resemblance to actor Anthony Hopkins—so much so that I half expected him to speak with a British accent.

"It sure does." Bob smiled, pressing my hand with callused palms.

"Staff tell me you're hoping to go home soon."

"Well, Cherí, I tell ya. It's like I told my family—if I'm gonna die, I wanna die at home in my own bed. Laura and me, we've lived in our house for fifty-seven years, and that's where I'm the most comfortable."

He and Laura exchanged glances.

"Sounds like a good plan to me. We'll do all we can to make it possible," I assured them both.

Bob's relative ease in talking about his impending death signaled an unusually deep level of acceptance. It was clear he and Laura were both straight shooters. No need to tiptoe around with these two.

"Hopefully, things will go just the way you want them to," I said. "Whatever happens, please know I'm available for you and your family."

Bob sat up straighter. "Well, Cherí, I've told my wife and daughter I'm not afraid to die, and I don't want them to be too sad, either. At least not too sad for me. I know where I'm going when I die."

"I can see you have a real peace about all this," I said, impressed by his beaming confidence. It's rare enough when a patient can articulate how she or he feels about dying, but it's rarer still to encounter such absolute faith about "the other side."

"You seem to feel so … good about dying. What's your secret?" I ventured.

Bob responded without hesitation. "I've been given a great gift, a pretty … uh, powerful experience that's really changed me. It's made me okay with all this." He seemed eager to disclose more, and I was eager to hear more.

"Would you mind telling me about it, Bob?"

"Oh, Bob saw heaven!" Laura blurted, her own excitement getting the best of her. "He had a vision. And he's not even a religious guy! It's helped us all so much."

"Well, I did have a vision," Bob added with a chuckle. "Never thought I'd be one of those people, but I guess I am." He lay back against his pillow, closing his eyes.

"I'd love to hear about it," I said, smiling at the reference to "those people." Did Bob have a near-death experience? Like many in hospice settings, I'd heard about patients like him but hadn't directly encountered one. Until now.

Bob's eyes remained closed. "You tell her about it, honey. I'm getting a little bit tired."

When I hear "tired," that's usually my cue to exit. "I can come back later, Bob. I don't want to tire you out."

"Oh no, it's fine: I want you to hear about it! Laura was there, too, so she can tell you." With that, Bob pulled the sheet up over his shoulders and settled in for a nap.

Laura leaned in toward me. "First I have to say, Cherí, Bob has never been a religious man. Never. He never went to church with me or Kim, our daughter. Oh, maybe once in a while at Christmas or Easter. But he just wasn't into it."

Bob interrupted, his eyes still closed. "But I believe in God. I've always believed in God. I just never was a church person."

Laura began the story. "Bob was diagnosed with pancreatic cancer over three years ago. It went into remission but then it came back—bad—about a year ago. We were busy trying to deal with the cancer and then, six months ago, he woke up one morning not feeling good at all. He had chest pains." She took a deep breath. "I panicked and insisted we go to the emergency room. When we got there, his heart stopped!"

She shook her head slightly. "The nurses started rushing around, calling the doctors. They pushed me out to the waiting room. It was awful! I wasn't told what was going on."

Bob piped up. "I was totally out of it; I don't even remember getting to the hospital."

"Then, Cherí, they got Bob's heart going again. The doctors finally came out and told me how Bob almost died. All the chemo from the past treatments weakened his heart, and he went into cardiac arrest."

Her voice took on a reverential tone. "But while his heart was stopped, he went to heaven! You know like some people have talked about dying and going to heaven and then coming back?"

"Yes. Oh my goodness!"

"He was in the hospital for a week. But he didn't say anything to us about it. I think he wasn't sure if we'd believe him. But two weeks later, at home, he asked if he could go to church with Kim and me. I said, 'Bob you know it's not a holiday, right?'"

She chuckled. "He said he wasn't confused—he wanted to go."

"Well, we go to church and Bob leans over to Kim and says, 'Those altar candles are pretty, but there's a lot more light than that in heaven.' And Kim doesn't know what to make of that."

Laura laughed. "She told me all about it at home. So I just came out and asked Bob, what did he mean about there being more light? And Bob sits there at the table and tells us how the candles reminded him of the brilliant lights he saw everywhere when his heart stopped, and how they were like lanterns lining the streets, and that it was so beautiful." Her voice dropped to a whisper when she pronounced "so beautiful."

"And he said even though the lights were so much brighter than anything here, he could look right at them without hurting his eyes. And they seemed to lead on and on without end, so he could see the street going on for miles. He said he saw Jesus in the distance, and Jesus told him not to be afraid, and that everything would be okay."

Bob sat up, unable to hold back. "Christ was far down the street when I saw him. But even though he was far away, when he spoke to me I could hear him perfectly—like he was standing right next to me." Bob's eyes shone.

"Isn't that something?" Laura said, looking to see what I thought about it all.

"It surely is," I agreed.

Bob spoke again. "Ever since then I've been okay with dying. Strange to say, I'm almost looking forward to it. Laura probably don't want me to say that, but I know what's gonna happen. I'm so thankful I got to tell Laura and Kim about it so they don't waste too much time feeling sad for me."

"Now that Bob's so happy about seeing heaven," Laura added, "we're just trying to enjoy our time together and have some fun. I just wish he could've gone to church with me sooner."

"Aw, honey …"

"How can I get upset about him dying, Cherí? He says constantly he's going to be just fine, and me and Kim will be, too."

"It sounds like your whole family's had a wonderful gift," I said.

"We have, and it's made such a difference," Laura said. "I kinda feel bad for people who don't get to know for sure about heaven. But Bob knows, and he's ready to go."

༄ ༄ ༄

As it turned out, Bob was discharged from the IPU the next day, and was was able to spend another whole month at home with his family. What's more, he died quietly in the night, pain-free, with both Laura and Kim present.

Three months later, Laura attended our loss support group, demonstrating a quiet confidence and minimal sadness. She was far more peaceful than most of the other participants.

"I know I'm coming to the end of my own life pretty soon," she told the group. "I don't wish to die but I don't mind, either. I'm so looking forward to being with Bob again."

There could be many reasons why patients might be reluctant to share experiences like Bob's, even with their own loved ones. The near-death experience (NDE) phenomenon remains mysterious despite ongoing investigation by scientists and medical researchers. To complicate the picture, some individuals have reported NDE-like experiences in situations that were not life-threatening.

Origins aside, those who have experienced an NDE often demonstrate a greater capacity to live purposefully and serve others. Whatever Bob experienced certainly had a profound impact on the way he viewed his own death.

Personally, I have no trouble believing there are those who see, hear, and connect with something that for now is inexplicable. In the meantime, I'm grateful to have encountered Bob and Laura. Their story stays with me, and reminds me to listen and watch our patients more closely for hints of their own encounters with Mystery.

BEFORE YOU GO

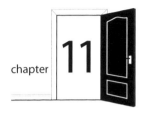

Carson

BEFORE YOU GO

Close to Home

The way we deal with loss shapes our capacity to be present to life more than anything else.

Rachel Remen

Everything changes when a death involves you and yours. Or should I say, everything is the same? Those of us who work daily with the terminally ill often assume that one day, when we are faced with the death of our own loved one, we'll navigate the experience better than average. We assume we won't struggle with what so many others have struggled with—simply because we know what to expect.

Not so. What I've learned proves otherwise. When I or my end-of-life associates are the parent, spouse, son, daughter, sibling of the one who is dying, it turns out we're just like everyone else. Our self-predicted composure and understanding dissolve into the typical responses of fear, anxiety, and grief—the very same responses we've seen in so many others.

I was reminded of this essential truth one bitter-cold day in February when Carson Nettle appeared in my life. Carson was a retired geriatric psychologist who for many years had counseled elderly patients and their families in a Florida hospital.

That morning had been a slow one, when our receptionist poked her head into my office. "Hey, there's a man at the front desk with his wife," Alice announced. "His mother is in the IPU for pain control, and he's very upset. Could you talk to him, Cherí?"

"I'm free for the next hour or so," I told her, glancing at my calendar. "Tell him I'll be right there." I took a last swallow of coffee, stood up and smoothed the wrinkles in my skirt, and headed for the front desk.

Carson Nettle stood waiting anxiously. He appeared to be around 60, a very tall and fit man with striking good looks. A deep tan set off his curly white hair and blue eyes. He was dressed in an expensive suit and tie, and looked every bit the career professional he once was.

By contrast, his wife, Evie, sat in a nearby chair, looking relaxed and comfortable. She was short and chubby, with a pleasant face, and dressed casually in croc gardening shoes, khaki pants, and a splashy Hawaiian print blouse. She gave me a smile as I approached.

The three of us exchanged introductions and shook hands. "So, Carson," I began, "I understand you'd like to talk about your mother?"

"Um, yes. My mom was just brought here and, well, I guess I'm having a hard time with it all."

"I'm free to talk with you for this next hour, if you like." I said. "Why don't we go somewhere more private? If you think it's okay, we could go back to your mom's room."

"Sure, that's fine. Mom's asleep and pretty out of it anyway."

We made our way past the front entrance and down the hall to his mother's room. Helen Nettle lay sleeping peacefully. Once a tall, athletic, and muscular woman, she had reached the end of a precipitous decline. Her frail, 93-year-old body under the white sheet looked to be that of a 10-year-old. Only her head and shoulders showed over the covers.

I leaned over the bed rail and gently patted the old woman's shoulder, whispering, "Hello, Helen."

Evie stepped up beside me and said in a low voice, "Mom just had her 93rd birthday last week. She really, really loved gardening, you know? Right up until last year she was still working in her own garden. Pretty amazing."

"Pretty amazing," I agreed.

"She loved it in Florida—just loved her flowers! She kept things growing all year round." Evie sighed with appreciation. "I'm not sure she'd be very happy with us if she knew we brought her back to cold, cold Wisconsin," she chuckled.

Carson said nothing but kept a close watch over his mother.

"Why don't we have a seat?" I suggested.

The three of us settled into the overstuffed chairs that filled the corner of Helen's large room. Carson and Evie sat across from me.

"Now, how can I help?" I asked, crossing my legs and settling back into my chair.

"Well, I'm a retired psychologist," Carson began, his tone suddenly direct and formal. "For most of my practice I worked in a hospital and specialized in the mental health of older adults. So I often worked with patients who eventually died."

"And here you are," I smiled, inviting him to put aside his professional persona.

He quickly dodged the invitation. "Twelve years ago Evie and I moved my mom down to Florida. She was still in really good health, and we had the resources to pay for a nice assisted living apartment near us. My sisters had done so much for her—it was my turn."

"What a gift for your mom and sisters," I said.

Carson only nodded. "My plan was, we would take care of mom and then she'd just die one day when her time came. I guess I never really thought about her lingering in a helpless state."

"So now here you are," I said again, "but maybe things aren't going quite the way you expected." It seemed Carson was caught up inside the same urgent scene he'd only experienced as an outsider. Where was the script for this?

"Mom lingering in pain was definitely not a part of the plan," he said with a note of surprise, as if registering a key insight. "Back when we moved her to Florida, I saw the situation as pretty straightforward. I had an idea of a treatment plan. Obviously I never wrote it down. It was more in my own mind. Whew!" He exhaled deeply. "I guess I just never saw this coming."

"And now you're dealing with the reality," I said gently.

"Exactly," Carson said with sudden clarity. "She's not a client, she's my mother dying in her own way, and I have no way to control how this all goes. Wow! It's just hitting me now." He looked as if he'd literally been punched in the gut.

To give him some gathering time, I excused myself and got up to check on Helen. She was sleeping quietly, undisturbed by our conversation. Taking her hand, I stroked it for a few moments. This was my personal reminder that she, our patient, was in the room with us, and we needed to acknowledge and respect her presence, too.

I rejoined Carson and Evie. "Carson, you were saying how your mom's situation didn't fit with your expectations."

"No, not at all. A few months ago Mom took a turn for the worse and really declined. She's been pretty much out of it ever since, and just barely eating. The doctor said her heart's failing, and she doesn't have much time left. That's why we brought her back here. I wanted my sisters to have some time to say goodbye. I think …"

I interrupted gently. More thinking was not what we needed. "Carson," I said, "Is it possible you might have some unfinished business with your mom? Is that why this is so hard?"

"No, no—it's not that. I've always had a great relationship with her. Evie, too. Mom loved her like her own daughter." He looked warmly at Evie. "I was lucky. My whole family was great—both my parents were teachers—and I wanted to give something back. It's part of why I became a psychologist."

Carson fidgeted with his tie and shifted in his seat. He wanted to fall back on the professional script he knew best, and could not, or would not, move into his own pain.

"You know, in my practice, I helped a lot of families adjust to their parents' aging, especially if they had dementia. And I always thought I had a good understanding of how this goes. But now, I don't know ..." He paused, closing his eyes and pinching the bridge of his nose to help keep his composure.

"Oh, for Godsake!" Carson blurted. "She's 93 years old; I know she can't live forever!" The controlled professional was crashing into the son about to lose his mother.

When he couldn't go on, Evie reached over and began to rub his back with a tender expression on her face, as if to say, *There now, that's what we've been waiting for.*

Clearing my throat, I said quietly, "She's your mother, Carson, and you've loved her so very much, for so long. Of course, you don't want to let her go."

We sat as silence filled the room. Suddenly Carson slumped forward and began to sob, softly at first but then uncontrollably. His shoulders shook as his heavy grief welled up from the depths.

I thought I'd never seen a man cry with such intensity.

His release was so powerful that I had to struggle to keep my own feelings in check. Maybe Evie did, too. Still, we kept silent as she continued rubbing Carson's back, gently and rhythmically. This woman's extraordinary sweetness was something special. She knew instinctively how to support her husband. It may have been mostly a generational thing, I know, but it was moving to see.

After a few moments, Evie reached over to the box of Kleenex on the end table, pulled out two tissues, and handed them to Carson. He looked up, red-faced from crying, and took them. "I can't let her go yet," he said, blowing his nose without embarrassment. "I guess I'm just not ready to say goodbye."

Helen did not linger much longer, to her children's great relief. She never regained consciousness and died peacefully in her sleep. Perhaps it was her final gift to them—the timing and manner of her passing a last gracious gesture. In any case, it's a scenario we see play out so often in hospice. With all three of her children gathered by her side, Helen had permission to take her leave. In the same way, the final ease with which she passed gave Carson and his sisters permission to let go.

"I guess I'm just not ready to say goodbye." Someone, somewhere, echoes Carson's lament every single moment of every day. I know this, but today it's a feeling that haunts my own life. The reason is my younger brother, Garth.

Two long years ago, Garth was diagnosed with colon cancer. He was only in his forties, with a wife and two teenage sons—a whole life! We all prayed liked crazy for his recovery. After undergoing surgery and chemotherapy, Garth went into remission, to our great joy.

A few months later, he had to undergo another assessment. As I was driving home after work, musing about what the doctors might find, my cell phone rang. I pounced. Maybe they had the results already.

"It's mom, Cherí."

"What's up, Mom? How's Garth doing?"

I caught my mother's hesitation in the smallest pause. It

said, *Brace yourself!* For sure, it was bad news. The cancer was not only back, it had metastasized to Garth's liver and maybe a couple other places. "We just don't know yet."

I pulled over to the curb and sat for a good cry. My brother was dying after all—my bold, bright, big-hearted, incorrigibly funny little brother. *No ... No ... I have no energy to deal with this—It's too much.* My tears spilled down my face. Out loud I spoke those three famous words: "It's not fair!"

For the next several days I functioned on autopilot. Each night after work, all that I'd done that day dropped away. I'd climb into my car—my sanctuary on wheels—and sit there for long moments staring out the windshield. Emotional exhaustion had replaced my usual "good tired" feeling at day's end. In its place my brain burned with a banner question: *Why this? Why now?*

Eventually I'd notice my hand turning the key in the ignition. Thank goodness the car knew its way home.

Those were rough days, all right. Since then, my expectations have been upended once more. At this writing, my brother's cancer has again gone into remission. This time I try not to be overly optimistic, knowing things could change in a heartbeat. I'm just grateful he and I have the opportunity to say what needs saying to each other. We have the luxury of a long goodbye.

Meanwhile, I cannot easily pull on my professional "cloak of invisibility" these days. Nor do I want to. If need be, I'll simply close my office door for quiet, tearful moments after my patient and family visits are over.

I know I'm not alone in this. Renowned hospice advocate Rachel Remen, author of *Kitchen Table Wisdom*, disputes the notion that those of us who work in hospice can remain untouched by the suffering and loss we see every day. She says it's like "expecting to be able to walk through water without getting wet."

Of course, the same truth applies to every one of us. As the old saw goes: Nobody gets out of this life alive. Nobody escapes getting wet sooner or later. It is my deep hope that you have taken these twelve stories to heart. And that, before you go, you will take good care to open your gifts. Say what you need to say. Learn to let go. Arrive at some peace. We are all closer to home than we know.